HOLISTIC MEDICINE

Harmony of   Body   Mind   Spirit

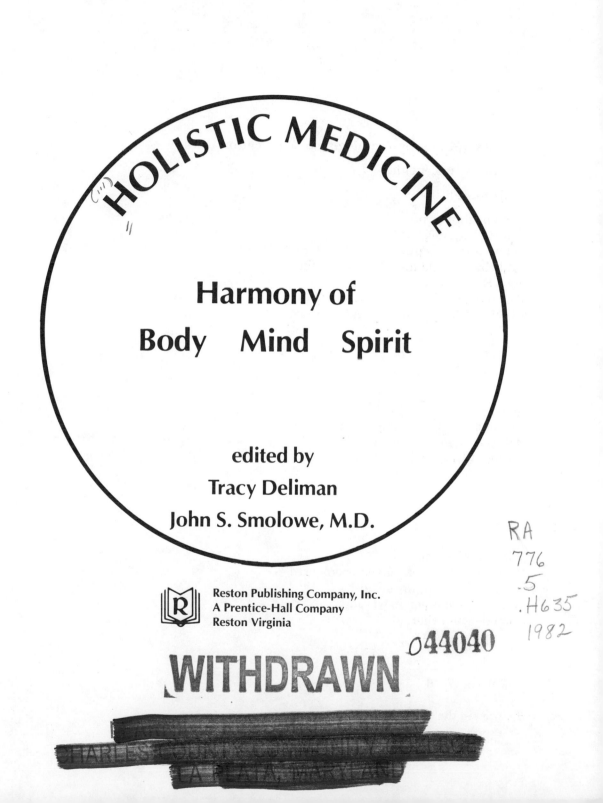

HOLISTIC MEDICINE

Harmony of
Body　Mind　Spirit

edited by

Tracy Deliman

John S. Smolowe, M.D.

Reston Publishing Company, Inc.
A Prentice-Hall Company
Reston Virginia

Library of Congress Cataloging in Publication Data

Main entry under title:

Holistic medicine.

 Bibliography: p.
 Includes index.
 1. Health.   2. Mind and body.   3. Holistic
medicine.   I. Deliman, Tracy.   II. Smolowe,
John S.
RA776.5.H635   613   82-3807
ISBN 0-8359-2844-6   AACR2

10   9   8   7   6   5   4   3   2   1

Printed in the United States of America.

To Mom and Dad and Ramon
Tracy

To Kitty, for singing
John

We have been trained to think of patterns, with the exception of those of music, as fixed affairs. It is easier and lazier that way but, of course, all nonsense. In truth, the right way to begin to think about the pattern which connects is to think of it as primarily (whatever that means) a dance of interacting parts and only secondarily pegged down by various sorts of physical limits and by those limits which organisms characteristically impose.

Gregory Bateson, *Mind and Nature*, 1979

CONTENTS

FOREWORD

A healthy life is still the unrealized hope of millions, even in the most developed societies. In addition to those diseases, injuries, and genetically transmitted conditions that modern medicine has not yet been able to treat effectively, contemporary industrial society itself creates health problems.

Pollution of water and air, stressful working and living environments, and poor nutrition affect the lives of people at every economic level. Further, some aspects of contemporary life—indiscriminate violence, alienation, erratically changing communities—undermine the gains of social programs designed to promote the public well being.

In recent years, the self-help movement in medicine, nutrition, rehabilitation, psychology, and related fields has sensitized the public to the importance of the *interrelationship* of physical, mental, and social factors in the improvement of health. This integrative, holistic trend has been most often connected with alternative health services and education. More recently, this trend is seen as moving parallel to, perhaps part of, a larger process now emerging world-wide.

In nations throughout the world, there is a growing recognition that individuals, societies, and the entire planet are vitally connected, not so much politically as organically. We see the necessity of feeding our expanding world population, and we have access to world-wide communications and travel. We have seen our Earth from space and we are facing the ominous knowledge that we have the power to either preserve or destroy our species. Like a person whose medical and self-examination reveals the need for a new approach to living if health is to be improved, our entire planetary society is slowly becoming aware of its precarious state of health and the need to change it.

The key word in this complex interaction of person, society, and planet is "awareness"—an awareness that we as individuals are parts of the whole and are responsible for all of it. This awareness may come from simply knowing ourselves and our world better. Sometimes it results from working with our own and others' suffering, and other times it comes from sharing great joy.

The authors of this book offer ideas, theories, practical guidance, techniques, and methods of everyday practice intended to help us cultivate awareness. Their contributions appear here as parts of an overall framework for a holistic approach to individual and social health. Behind their work is an understanding they share in common: it is essential to respect one's life and care for it; to learn to live *with* life rather than against it; to enjoy it and appreciate its wonders; to share it with others. This approach in its most direct form is simply an attitude of compassion toward ourselves and others. It is a natural human basis for living a life that is healthy and whole.

Miles A. Vich
Editor
Journal of Transpersonal Psychology

ACKNOWLEDGEMENTS

I have many people to thank for their role in this undertaking. For support and advice throughout, I thank Miles Vich, Jack Downing, and Henry Dakin at the Washington Research Center. I would also like to thank several colleagues and friends who shared ideas that entered into the shaping of this book: Dale Peterson, Chantal Decleve, Ayse and Wells Whitney, David Cole, Bob Albrecht, Mildred Dittmar, and my husband, Ramon Zamora.

I especially thank all the contributors to this volume for their willingness to cast their material by our framework and for their contribution to our growth and, ultimately, to the growth of others.

Tracy Deliman

I would like to thank:

My wife, Joellen Werne, for teaching me about closeness; for being warm, assertive, and flexible; and for being a great mother to Laura Danielle;

Jack Downing, who is light-hearted and available and who taught me about pioneers and settlers;

Rudolph Ballentine, for sharing his early doubts about writing;

Joan Wager, for being a big sister who knows just what I like to study;

Arthur Kidd, for showing me that reflexology works and for being Arthur;

My mother, who inspired my vision of walking into the room and diagnosing clients' problems without technology;

My father, for supporting my sense of my own direction;

Anson, who was a big brother as long as he could be;

Matthew and Betsie Haar, Don Hansen, and Lynn and Julian Gorodsky, for being my friends;

Randy Charlton, Hillary Greene, Jim Bugental and, again, Jack Downing, for referring us to contributors;

Miles Kastendieck, who was a great English teacher;

Al Bauman, for being a *mensch*;

My clients and students for engaging with me, for teaching me, and for giving me examples for the book;

The many others who've given me ideas and support along the way, including Heather and Jay Ogilvy, Jack Kornfield, John Beletsis, Ed Weiss, Susan Merrill, Herb Shepard, Irene Garrow, Naomi Werne, Emmett Miller, Jonathan Krown, Alice Sargent, Ginger Lapid, Marshall Edelson, Dan Levinson, Ken Keniston, and Gloria, Norm, and Joanie.

John S. Smolowe

Grateful acknowledgement is made for permission to reprint from the following works:

Diet & Nutrition, A Holistic Approach, by Rudolph Ballentine (Honesdale, PA: Himalayan International Institute, 1978). Permission granted by Rudolph Ballentine, M.D., and the Himalayan International Institute.

Breathing, The ABC's, by Carola H. Speads (New York: Harper & Row, 1978). Permission granted by Carola Speads and Harper & Row.

Holism and Evolution, by Jan Christiaan Smuts (New York: Macmillan Publishing Company, 1926). Permission granted by the estate of Jan Christiaan Smuts.

CONTRIBUTOR BIOGRAPHIES

Rudolph Ballentine, M.D.   Dr. Ballentine is Director of the Combined Therapy Program at the Himalayan International Institute in Honesdale, Pennsylvania, and coordinates a network of outpatient clinics. His practice integrates nutrition, meditation, Ayurvedic medicine, homeopathy, and psychotherapy. He is author of *Diet & Nutrition, A Holistic Approach*, co-author of *Science of Breath*, and *Yoga and Psychotherapy*.

Al Bauman.   Mr. Bauman is a professional non-therapist. He was trained as a musician and in theatre, and he spent 30 years as a concert pianist, teacher of music at eastern universities, and as actor and director of children's theatre. After meeting Wilhelm Reich in 1948, Mr. Bauman applied Reich's concepts to the training of musicians, dancers, and artists. For 10 years, he lived in Synanon, developing and directing an educational system for children and adults. More recently, at the invitation of a group of psychotherapists, Mr. Bauman has been training people in Reich's work through a continuing Workshop of Expression. He is in private practice in Santa Barbara, California.

Tracy Deliman.   Ms. Deliman is an anthropologist, with focus in medical anthropology, and a research associate at Washington Research Center in San Francisco. She has done fieldwork in Brazil and San Francisco studying different medical beliefs and systems. Her research interests combine medical anthropology, transpersonal psychology, and spiritual healing. She is author of numerous freelance articles in general subjects.

Jack Downing, M.D.   Dr. Downing was trained at the Menninger Clinic in Topeka, Kansas, and with Fritz Perls, Oscar Ichazo, and Ida Rolf. He directed the San Mateo County Mental Health System in California, founded the Center for the Healing Arts in New York City in 1976, and was a founding member of the Gestalt Institute of San Francisco, and of the Arica Institute of New York City. Dr. Downing was a leader in the investigation of the social and individual implications of LSD therapy. He is author of *Dreams and Nightmares*; *Gestalt Awareness*; and *The Handbook of Community Mental Health*. He is now in private practice of comprehensive psychiatry, including rolfing, applied kinesiology, and neurolinguistic programming, in San Francisco.

Hector Goa, M.D.   Dr. Goa is a psychiatrist for children and adolescents. He teaches and practices in New York City. Dr. Goa's present interest is the significance of the family as a school for living.

Anna Halprin.   Ms. Halprin is founder and director of the San Francisco Dancers' Workshop and Director of the Tamalpa Institute of the Dancers' Workshop. She has developed a form of dance that is a powerful tool for integrating personal and artistic growth. She has done special workshops, performances, guest lectures, and public rituals for many organizations and conferences throughout the country and abroad. Ms. Halprin is author of *Movement Ritual I*, *Collected Writings I and II*, and *A School Comes Home*, and her work is documented in films, videotapes and articles.

Daria Halprin-Khalighi.   Ms. Halprin-Khalighi is co-director of the Tamalpa Institute of the San Francisco Dancers' Workshop. She is a movement and gestalt therapist who integrates creativity, dance, gestalt, and visualization experiences in her work. She has participated as guest presenter in several conferences and has appeared in films, including *Jerusalem Files* and *Zabriskie Point*.

Robert K. Hall, M.D.   Dr. Hall is a psychiatrist and teacher. He was trained in gestalt by Fritz Perls, in structural integration by Ida Rolf, and in polarity therapy by Randolph Stone. He is a co-founder of the Lomi School in Marin, California, and of the San Francisco Gestalt Institute. He is currently chairman of the Sonoma Institute faculty and is in private practice in body-oriented therapy. Dr. Hall teaches throughout the United States and Europe and trains therapists in the somatic awareness disciplines.

Albert Kreinheder, Ph.D.   Dr. Kreinheder is a clinical psychologist and Jungian analyst, and is past president and director of training of the Carl G. Jung Institute in Los Angeles, California. He has written articles on dreams, creativity, and the individuation process. His present interest is in the use of symbolic imagery as a healing bridge between the body and the psyche.

Emmett M. Miller, M.D.   Dr. Miller's practice and research incorporates techniques of psychophysiological control. He has integrated Eastern and Western disciplines to produce techniques for reducing stress and tension and to aid in relaxation imagery and facilitation of the healing response. He developed applications of these techniques for use in self-motivation, effective communication patterns, actualization of a desirable self-image, and enhancement of wellness. Dr. Miller leads lay and professional workshops in Menlo Park, California.

James Thomas Pope.   Mr. Pope was graduated from Echerd College with a Bachelor of Arts degree in literature, and he is an associate of Lomi School in Marin, California. He has studied mind/body therapy extensively with Dr. Robert K. Hall, and is a life-long student of movement and theater arts. Presently, he lives on the northern California coast, where he incorporates touch, verbal communication, and body movement in his private practice and teaching.

John Smolowe, M.D.   Dr. Smolowe is a psychiatrist who incorporates awareness, movement, imagery, and breathing into his practice in Menlo Park, California. He is an associate member of the Gestalt Institute of San Francisco, a faculty member of Pacific Graduate School of Psychology, and a clinical faculty member of the Stanford University Department of Psychiatry.

Carola H. Speads.   Ms. Speads is a teacher and practitioner in the field of physical re-education, with specialization in breathing. She trained and worked first in Germany, where she practiced in close collaboration with Elsa Gindler, and now works in New York at the Studio of Physical Re-education. She is the author of *Breathing, The ABC's.*

David S. Walther, D.C.   Dr. Walther is Director of the Chiropractic Health Center of Pueblo, Colorado, and has used applied kinesiology since its inception in 1964. He is Vice-Chairman of the International College of Applied Kinesiology, and he developed the format of teaching used in the organization. Dr. Walther lectures throughout the United States and Europe and is the author of *Applied Kinesiology—The Advanced Approach in Chiropractic* (1976), 10 volumes of *Applied Kinesiology Programmed Instruction*, (1977–78), *Applied Kinesiology Flow Chart* (1980), *Applied Kinesiology, Volume I—Basic Procedures and Muscle Testing* (1981).

Ayse Whitney.   Ms. Whitney was raised in the Middle East and holds an M.A. in social psychology from the University of Strasbourg, France. She has pursued a meditation practice for 25 years and has made an extensive study of Eastern and Western religious philosophies. She started teaching meditation and the Yoga of Light shortly after her arrival in the United States in 1966. Today, she is the head of the White Eagle Yoga Center in

Menlo Park, California, where she continues her teaching and also practices as an intuitive counselor and astrologer.

Jack Worsley, Dr.Ac.   Dr. Worsley is Professor and Master of traditional Chinese acupuncture; Founder-President of the College of Traditional Chinese Acupuncture, United Kingdom; Honorary Professor of the Department of Oriental Medicine, Won Kwang University, Korea; Vice-President of the World Academic Society of Acupuncture; and Honorary President of Compagnonnage de Acupuncture Traditionelle. Professor Worsley has lectured throughout the United States, Europe, and the Far East on aspects of traditional Chinese medicine and acupuncture. He is the author of *Traditional Chinese Acupuncture, Volume I—Meridians and Points*; *Is Acupuncture for You?*; *Acupuncturists' Therapeutic Pocket Book*; and *The Meridians of Ch'i Energy: Point Reference Guide* and set of charts.

HOLISTIC MEDICINE
Harmony of Body Mind Spirit

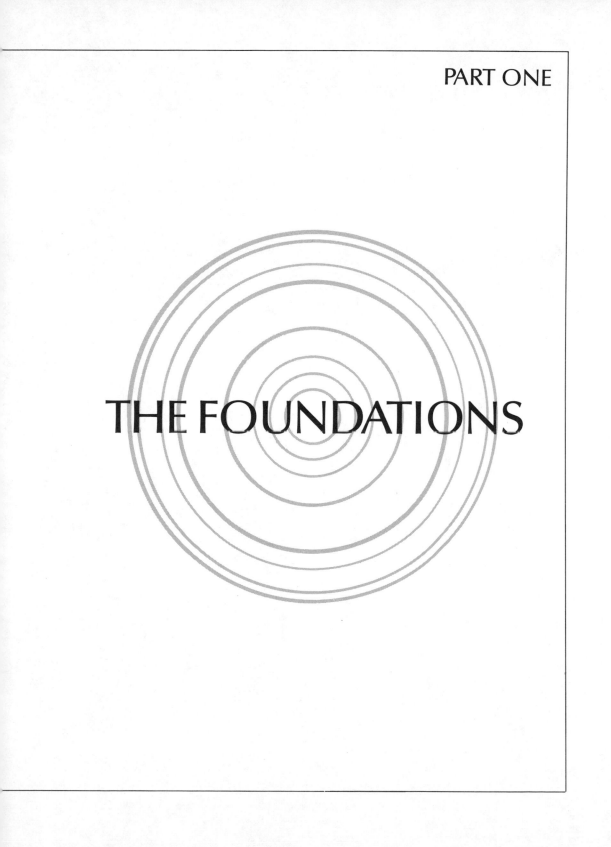

PART ONE

THE FOUNDATIONS

INTRODUCTION

TRACY DELIMAN

Holism—a theory that the universe and especially living nature is correctly seen in terms of interacting wholes (as of living organisms) that are more than the mere sum of elementary particles.

Webster's New Collegiate Dictionary

For all its recent success, holistic medicine lacks a unifying framework. Although the growth toward a holistic approach over the last 20 years has been purposeful, holism itself has been unclearly conceived of by its practitioners and recipients, producing a diverse understanding of the holistic process. The central focus has been on treatments, rather than on the client. To be unified, holistic practice must be focused on the client and should be carried out with a consistent theoretical framework. The editors of this volume have come to the conclusion that the ideal in holistic practice is to be integrative, to form a more complete, coordinated whole of the client. This usually means being comprehensive about the client and including all aspects of the client in diagnosis and treatment. In holistic medicine, a person can be viewed realistically as a whole organism with many dimensions that function interdependently. These dimensions represent different views of the whole and different functions of the whole. The dimensions are sensitively integrated into the functioning of the whole; change in one dimension effects change in others. The nature of these dimensions and their relationships to one another can be understood and used effectively in treatment.

These beliefs—that there are many dimensions to a person, that these dimensions are integrated into the whole, and that the approach should be comprehensive—form the basis of the multidimensional approach. It is our purpose in this book to establish a theoretical framework leading to a viable approach in holistic medical care.

IDEAS IN HOLISM

Some of the kernel ideas of holistic philosophy date from antiquity and have undergone refinement over time, while others are thoroughly modern. The notion of the soundness of mind and body together and the belief in both the natural cause of disease and the existence of a natural healing force are quite old. The concepts of balance or balance-seeking and energy also have a long and widespread history. Most central to holistic philosophy are the ideas of wholeness or one-

5

ness of entities and the existence of functional interdependence among parts and wholes. Lastly, the idea of client responsibility has little mention in history but is of great importance in modern holism.

Perhaps the earliest germ of holistic thought lies in the classic Greek ideal of a sound mind in a sound body, an idea that has filtered down through the centuries. In the time of the ancient Greek physician Hippocrates, the father of modern medicine, disease was considered to be created by natural causes. Hippocrates believed that the physician's role was to assist nature's own healing force. His first interest was the patient, not the disease itself, and his concern was with the body as a whole. Symptoms served as indicators of the status of the patient, rather than as a basis of classification.

During the European Renaissance, humanists in medicine reinterpreted many Hippocratic ideas. Additionally, their efforts to interpret "miracles" rationally resulted in a greater insight into the role of psychological factors in disease; "imagination" was recognized as a factor in the genesis and cure of many diseases.

In the mid 1800s, Claude Bernard, a French physiologist and biochemist, developed the concept of homeostasis or balance seeking. He theorized that an internal environment existed as a mediator between the life of the organism and its external environment. The organism tends to maintain the composition of this environment so that, if the dynamic equilibrium is upset, reactions occur to restore the balance.

Physics, the other natural sciences, and philosophy accepted the separateness of matter, mind, and spirit until the middle to late nineteenth century, when certain individuals began discovering interconnections among these elements of the universe. Darwin's theory of evolution influenced the concept of holism in two ways: first, by showing an interrelatedness between an organism and its environment, and then by indicating a responsive flexibility of the species in nature. By the early twentieth century, the newly developed theory of relativity in physics showed an interdependence of time and space and redefined the structural character of the universe to one of greater complexity and interrelatedness. These developments had begun to undermine the prevalent physical materialist philosophy that was responsible for a mechanistic view of nature and a rigid concept of causation.

These ideas were crystalized into a theory of holism in the 1920s by Jan Christiaan Smuts, a South African statesman and philosopher who, in fact, originated the term "holism." Smuts realized rigid materialism could no longer explain nature, and thus, he deepened his inquiry into the idea of "wholes" in nature. He ultimately arrived at the concept of holism. (Smuts' view of holism is explained in greater detail in the next chapter.)

Beginning in the 1930s, the philosophical schools of phenomenology and existentialism achieved widespread influence in Western culture. The teaching of the German existentialist, Martin Heidegger, promoted the idea of being-in-the-world, where the human and the world are considered as one encompassing whole. Human existence cannot be separated from the world as subject and object, but instead they are together one inextricable, fundamental category. This marks a substantial divergence from the dualism permeating Western thought for the past three centuries. Also within existentialist thought, Jean Paul Sartre, the French dramatist and philosopher, developed the idea of personal responsibility.

In psychology, beginning in the 1950s, Abraham Maslow promoted the idea of self-actualization, thus furthering the concept of personal responsibility. In self-actualization, the individual assumes greater power in realizing his or her potential and direction in the world. Fritz Perls, R.D. Laing, and others also promoted personal responsibility. Thus, the focus in psychology became one of personal growth, moving away from the psychopathology model.

Social changes during the 1960s, such as human liberation movements, civil rights, and self-help trends, also inspired modern holistic thought. Among these was the interest in self-actualization, which translated to client responsibility in the sphere of health care. Also prevalent in the sixties and seventies was a re-emergence of the personal, self-directed search for mystical and religious meaning in life, involving meditation and other disciplines that seek inner knowledge. Through these experiences, people began recognizing the spiritual part of human nature and the desire to nurture this dimension. Deeper levels of religious experience lead to realization of the wholeness or oneness of living entities.

In recent years, the influence of the East has been a major factor in the shaping of holistic concepts and practices. In the late 1960s, the United States increased trade and commercial relations with Eastern countries, notably India and Pakistan, and later with China. The climate became one of increased acceptance and curiosity about cultural differences. Westerners began wearing Eastern clothes and using Eastern furniture and material items, and many people incorporated disciplines such as yoga, meditation, and oriental martial arts into their daily lives. The re-opening of formal political relations between the United States and China in 1971 was followed by a surge of interest in acupuncture and Chinese medicine among medical professionals and laypeople.

Although the Chinese explanations of acupuncture and medicine are vastly different from concepts in Western thought, a few are clearly recognizable and are pertinent to holistic theory. *Yin* and *yang* represent forces of opposites, in or seeking a state of balance. They are conceived of as a unit that is present within all living organisms. Chinese medical theory also emphasizes the organic or functional interrelationships between parts and wholes through the belief that the energy level and status of one part of the body affects other parts and, thus, the whole. Additionally, the Chinese concept of *ch'i*, or energy, influences the holistic idea of a vital life force in the human being.

◎ THE NATURE OF THE HOLISTIC APPROACH

Many of the therapies in holistic health have come from different parts of the world and are entirely new to Western culture. Others developed in the United States. The few that became established in the United States often underwent redefinition and further development before they were incorporated into the holistic idiom. The evolved practices are sometimes referred to as "alternative" because they are usually seen as alternatives to conventional medical practices. By now, the names of many of these interventions are known to the general public: acupuncture, rolfing, meditation, shiatsu, bodywork, homeopathy, herbology, dance therapy, applied kinesiology, chiropractic therapy, imagery and visualization therapy, psychosynthesis, psychic healing, and so forth. The ways in which these therapies are used vary.

In its usual eclectic form, holistic practice means collecting a wide range of information about a person, drawing a series of generalizations from this information, and then selecting a therapy. From the diversity of techniques available, the practitioner or client selects one or several therapies that appear to be the most appropriate for a given complex of symptoms or one believed to be the best all-around therapy.

This approach can sometimes be effective in bringing about a cure. The approach is not comprehensive or systematic in its assessment of the person, however. It does not attempt to discern the status of different aspects of the person, such as breathing, movement, structure, or spiritual and emotional wellness, nor does it attempt to discover how certain of these parts are interrelating and affecting the health of the person.

Combining several techniques in an eclectic approach or using a single innovative technique, such as rolfing or shiatsu, does not necessarily make one's treatment holistic. Obviously, therapies by themselves cannot be holistic. The entire *approach itself* must be holistic: this includes a way of viewing, an attitude, and a general diagnostic procedure, as well as therapeutic practices.

Multidimensional holism is a new proposal in the principles and practices of holistic medicine. Within this framework, the person is seen as a whole comprised of dimensions that interact with one another, such as movement, structure, breath, spirit, and so forth. These dimensions are so intimately and sensitively interrelated that change in one part brings about shifts in other parts. Illness, then, is a disturbance of the unified functioning of the whole and not just an isolated cause or effect.

Using the purest form of the holistic model, it could be argued that one should not attempt to analyze the person into parts at all; if the human being is a totally integrated entity, the division is not possible. In a sense, this is absolutely true. But, in approaching the individual diagnostically, it may be necessary to take aspects of the person and examine them separately. The divisions we make here are functional. Also, most of these dimensions can be experienced and are not simply theoretical. In making divisions, we have tried not to lose sight of the integrity of the person.

The *nutritional dimension* is defined by what a person does with his or her diet, not by specific rules of nutrition. The definition includes the dimension's relationship to awareness, energy, personal responsibility, emotions, and bodily sensation. The *structural dimension* we consider to be the arrangement of muscles and bones, including posture, muscle tension, and flexibility. *Movement* is the body in motion, including expressiveness, creativity, and moods. We consider *emotion* as an internally felt response and a coloration of the outside world. It is a capacity that can return the person to equilibrium, rather than a driving characteristic or quality separate from the person. The *breathing dimension* is inhalations, exhalations, and pauses, and it also involves breathing sensations, kinesthetic sense, muscle tonus, and circulation. It includes the ability of the breath to adjust naturally and involuntarily to different situations.

The *symbolic dimension* includes personal symbols that can be used as a means of learning about oneself but not necessarily universal symbols translated at an individual level. Through the *sensory/imagery dimension*, the person receives and processes information from the external and internal environment. These senses are touch, taste, smell, hearing, and vision mainly. Perception and imagery are two ways of sensing; perception corresponds to an external object, while imagery does not. We see *awareness* as the capacity to notice things, such as subtle or gross aspects of oneself, including bodily sensation, emotions, thought, spirituality, and energy. Awareness can be clear or hazy, continuous or broken. *Energy* we consider as the vital life force of a person, a liveliness that the human being contains and radiates, which changes in varying states of health and illness.

The *spiritual dimension* is the soul, which permeates all parts of the person and comprises our efforts for developing higher consciousness and religious or mystical qualities. The *meridians* comprise a system of energy running on known pathways throughout the body—a set of energy patterns for the whole of the person. Other dimensions, such as the interpersonal, cardiovascular, and mental, could also be included in this multidimensional approach.

The attitude in multidimensional holism is one of great receptiveness and flexibility. It is compassionate. It requires getting to know each person as a unique individual, looking at that person's life openly and including every aspect of personal history, sensibility, physicality, energy, and motivation. An individual may have an entire complex of symptoms that appear to be unrelated to one another or to the illness. But all symptoms are at least broadly meaningful and can be seen as clues to the status of any of the dimensions, as well as to certain aspects or causes of the condition. The whole symptom complex is taken into consideration in the diagnostic procedure, no matter which dimension of the person is favored.

People who use this multidimensional approach know, intuitively or consciously, many of the ways in which the human dimensions interrelate, and they use the interrelations to advantage in therapy. It may mean, for example, interplaying the emotional dimension with the movement dimension until an emotional discomfort becomes clear and controllable. Or it may mean enhancing the awareness dimension in relation to the nutritional dimension so that one becomes keenly aware of the effects of specific nutrients.

The authors contributing to this book include in their approach to healing several, and sometimes all, of the dimensions we described earlier. Typically, they begin their works with a concentration on one dimension or another. They discuss relationships of one dimension to others and then describe their methods of working. This format is basic to the guidelines we developed for the authors to follow in building their chapters. These guidelines were designed so that the authors' material would illustrate our conception of multidimensional holism. They are as follows:

1. Describe the dimension, and consider what healthy or normal functioning is in this dimension and what impairment is.

Consider what certain kinds of impairment indicate in the health of the individual.

2. What assumptions do practitioners that work with this dimension have?

3. Where do you look in the human being to measure function (for example, posture, muscular functioning, breath, pulses, etc.), and what variables do you measure or assess?

4. What interventions (therapies or modes of treatment) do you use to produce change in this dimension, and how do you recognize improvement? How well does improvement in this dimension extend to other dimensions and to the whole person? Please include examples.

5. To what extent does the practitioner heal the client; to what extent does the practitioner train the client to heal himself or herself? What might the client do to maintain a balanced healthy system?

6. Mention at least briefly the major types of interventions that emphasize this dimension, and discuss one in more depth, including diagnosis and treatment. If you can, note how findings and interventions in this dimension correlate with symptoms and results in other dimensions.

7. Please mention any limitations in working with this dimension alone for attaining total well-being and any limitations in using your chosen intervention.

Most of the authors followed the guidelines, except those who were required by the particular nature of their theory and practice to reinterpret some of the guidelines—specifically, Jack Worsley, Ayse Whitney, and Albert Kreinheder. In the resulting chapters, most of the authors exemplify the multidimensional approach: they relate one dimension to at least a few others and base their treatment on that relationship. A few of the authors do not intentionally draw relations among the dimensions.

In examining these dimensions, many questions are answered and still others arise. Are the meridians real pathways of energy, or do they comprise a construct tied to Chinese medical theory and acupuncture technique? Is the spiritual dimension the same as one's religious sense, or is it a parallel dimension, like structure or movement? Is awareness a capacity we can develop, like a musical or artistic talent, or is it fully a dimension, too?

The methods used by Anna Halprin and Daria Halprin-Khalighi in the movement dimension assess broad divisions of the person—physical, mental, emotional, and spiritual. In the physical area, the

goal is to learn to sense the body in movement. In the emotional area, it is to identify one's condition and break through old patterns. In the mental area, it is to learn to accumulate resources and to plan and evaluate creatively. In the spiritual area, the goal is to experience the connection between oneself and the whole of human nature. Halprin and Halprin-Khalighi consider that movement involves all parts of the person as a whole, including energy, emotion, thought, and images. They ask the client to draw a picture of his or her own body and then to "dance" the picture; thus, imagery and movement are connected. Areas of weakness and dysfunction are manifested in the way a person moves.

David Walther begins his work by considering the structural dimension. He makes one-to-one correlations between one dimension and another, using applied kinesiology as the diagnostic tool. A phenomenon in the musculoskeletal dimension indicates health or illness in an organ. When an organ or dimension of a person is not functioning well, a corresponding group of muscles is weakened. Weakening is a correlate of the dysfunctional condition of an organ, while testing the muscles for strength tells the applied kinesiologist which organs are dysfunctional.

The meridians, described by Jack Worsley, are viewed as pathways of vital energy, each of which is connected with a major organ or dimension: stomach, lung, colon, kidneys, bladder, liver, gall bladder, heart, small intestine, circulation-sex, and triple-heater. Worsley assesses these areas by reading 12 pulses located at specific points on the wrists. Each pulse tells the state of organs or functions and the quality or quantity of life energy. The pulses are considered to be an actual part of the meridian complex. He assesses the mental and emotional areas through color, sound, smell, and personal and family history. Worsley develops a comprehensive picture of the client and determines a treatment strategy to treat every area needed to bring about a wholly healthy person.

In working with the nutritional dimension, Rudolph Ballentine defines health and nutrition in terms of an interrelationship between nutrients and awareness, not in terms of what is "right to eat." He integrates relaxation, meditation, breathing, yoga, Ayurvedic medicine, homeopathy, and counseling to approach the subtleties of what a person does with his or her diet. The purpose is to cultivate awareness in the person, thus increasing sensitivity to the body's signals about nutrients and eating habits. A process of self-study evolves, focusing on the interaction between the awareness and nutritional dimensions, enabling the person to make changes gradually.

The chapter by Robert Hall and James Thomas Pope shows the

same basic approach as Ballentine, but the focus is on awareness it-self, with the body as a tool for enhancing that awareness. They use the physical aspect of a problem area and develop awareness through it. Understanding the functioning of a body area and its interrela-tions to emotions and other faculties is taken to deeper levels through awareness exercises.

In the energy dimension, Al Bauman sees a general demeanor of the person, noticing where energy is concentrated, where it is lack-ing, and how it flows. If energy is in balance and flowing smoothly, says Bauman, the person has a sense of unity, movement is flexible and integrated, breathing is easy, and emotional expression is spon-taneous and full. Bauman uses massage, touch, breathing, or motion to increase or decrease the energy flow or to draw energy from one area to another.

Carola Speads relates breathing indirectly to many bodily proc-esses: muscle tone, circulation, organ functioning, moods, energy, and creativity. Through subtle breathing exercises, she focuses the breathing work on awareness of the self, of breathing and its effects on other dimensions, and on the ways people interfere with breath-ing. Speads relies on the person's body sense to develop the awareness, since sensations inform the person of the state of his or her breathing.

Emmett Miller also relates the sensory/imagery dimension indi-rectly to other dimensions. Imagery can be an indicator and determi-nant of emotional functioning, an influence on energy level and bod-ily functions, and an adjunct to creativity. Miller assesses the imaging ability by asking questions that would bring images to mind or by asking the person to picture certain situations or experiences. Imag-ery treatment may involve, for example, going within the body and visualizing it healing or changing. Healing in one area can lead to changes in other areas.

John Smolowe first defines the emotional dimension by itself. Then he connects it with other related dimensions: body, sensation, imagery, and energy. In this way, certain of the dimensions are explic-itly integrated. He considers constraint, exaggeration, and frag-mented emotional response as the mechanisms of emotional diffi-culty. For example, disengagement of the awareness part from the physical part can mean the person may not know that he or she is reacting to an emotional stimulus. Asking a client to notice effects of certain exercises or emotions on other dimensions clarifies the rela-tionship to those dimensions.

Ayse Whitney works with the spiritual dimension of her clients through yoga, meditation, chanting, breathing, massage, and coun-seling. She first defines spirituality by itself and then relates it to other dimensions, such as bodily sensations, emotions, and images. Clients are asked to take certain bodily positions in yoga. Then they sit with the sensations and reactions to see what happens to their mood and spirituality. This allows an exploration of the innermost spiritual, emotional, mental, and physical aspects of the person, developing awareness and integrating the person's spirituality with other dimensions.

In Albert Kreinheder's work, the personal symbolic system is used to teach a person what needs to be known about his or her whole self. A person can become more aware of the symbolic content of illness conditions and can understand the symbols to which attention should be given. In extensive encounters with symbols, a person gets deeper into the images and can advance toward healing. Attention is called to the necessity of personal changes and to areas of potential positive growth.

In the third section of the book, Hector Goa defines the key elements of a successful healing relationship in the holistic model. He stresses that therapy must be based on the development of human consciousness. The therapist must deal with the human being as a whole and must himself be continuously engaged in inner work. The therapist should relate his or her whole life with other lives and include himself or herself as part of the treatment. Maintaining a healthy balance between inner awareness and the outward encounter with the client allows sincerity and promotes interpersonal freedom, rather than dependency.

The chapter by Jack Downing discusses problems and ideal possibilities for the holistic health center. Rules are necessary, but they must be flexible according to the needs of people, says Downing. The center ought to tend all facets of the client and promote positive health. Downing applies holistic principles to the health-enhancing goals of the center: the center itself is comprised of parts functioning as a whole; the client is a part of the center and must be responsible. He elaborates further on the reciprocal nature of the client/center relationship.

We have intended the works in this book to form the basis of a multidimensional approach to healing. We hope that this work, along with the efforts of these practitioners and many others like them, lays the foundation for a unifying framework in holistic medicine. Early in our contact with these authors, when we invited them to contribute a chapter on a particular dimension, most asked the question, "How can I possibly talk about one dimension without also talking about the others?" Once involved in this approach, it is obvious that no one dimension can be isolated. By definition, each dimension connects to the others. The multidimensional approach addresses the many aspects of a person and is thus genuinely holistic. It is anticipated that this multidimensional approach will continue to be refined by these and the many other practitioners and laypeople who adopt it.

REFERENCES

Tracy Deliman. "The Integration of Acupuncture and Chinese Medicine into the American Medical System" (Master's thesis, San Francisco State University, 1978).

Martin Heidegger. *Being and Time* (New York: Harper & Row, 1962).

J.M.D. Olmsted. *Claude Bernard, Physiologist* (New York: Harper and Bros., 1938).

J.C. Smuts. *Holism and Evolution* (New York: Macmillan Publishing Company, 1926).

Jack R. Worsley. *Is Acupuncture for You?* (New York: Harper & Row, 1973).

THE ORIGINS
OF HOLISM

JAN CHRISTIAAN SMUTS

The concept of holism originated through a long series of intuitive and logical deductions about wholes in nature. Its creator, Jan Christiaan Smuts, was primarily a statesman only peripherally involved in science. His book, *Holism and Evolution*, is a penetrating examination of the interrelatedness of elements of the universe. It was published in 1926, at the height of his political career.

Of Dutch ancestry, Smuts was born a British subject in the Cape Colony of South Africa in 1870. He was educated at Cambridge in science, arts, and law and won numerous honors and awards. Upon his return to South Africa, Smuts entered immediately into politics. He was twice prime minister of South Africa, first during the 1920s and again from 1939 throughout the 1940s. Smuts fought the British for an independent and united South Africa. He was drawn into international affairs during World War I and was one of the principal progenitors of the League of Nations. Smuts was an accomplished statesman, though not a popular leader. He had a sophisticated mind and was enormously hardworking, but he had little patience with mediocrity and was not easily sociable.

Smuts read widely in philosophy, law, poetry, and science and apparently kept abreast of scientific developments and theories prevalent in his time. He was convinced that greater contact between science and philosophy would prove fruitful for both fields. He believed in a synthetic tendency in the universe and eventually conceived of holism as the principle that underlies this tendency and makes for the origin and progress of wholes in the universe.

Holism and Evolution centered on a discussion of matter, life, and mind within the contexts of various theories prevalent in the early 1900s. The first four chapters, summarized here, developed the theory of holism. (As an aside, Smuts spoke of "life" in much the same tone and context as we now speak of "spirit" or "soul.")

SYNOPSIS OF THE FIRST FOUR CHAPTERS

Matter, life, and mind are seen as quite separate from one another. The more advanced concepts of evolution, namely variation and natural selection, were major topics in Smuts' era, since Darwin's theory of evolution had gained wide acceptance in the late nineteenth and early twentieth centuries. Smuts contended that acceptance of evolution necessitated readjustment of views on matter, life, and mind. Specifically, he felt that acceptance of the origin of life structures from the inorganic means matter could no longer be viewed in the physical materialist, mechanical framework.

In Smuts' era, concepts in science and philosophy had narrowed to rigidity: ideas of interactions and connections were virtually precluded, and nature was viewed as inflexible and mechanical rather than fluid. Also, the concept of causation in nineteenth century science—that there could be no more in the effect than in the cause—made creativeness and real progress impossible. Smuts rethought these concepts into a view of the fundamental unity and continuity underlying matter, life, and mind. He saw the three as intimately connected parts in the same great process.

Smuts then noted that the theory of relativity was replacing Newtonian concepts of space and time, as a result of research into the relative character of all actual motion in the universe. The revolutionary discovery was the interdependence of time and space: any perception of space would vary with different dimensions of time, and time and space together formed the units of reality. Extensions of this theory gave a definite structural character to the universe, accounting for previously unexplained phenomena.

Smuts proposed that the aspect of structure placed matter in a new perspective. With the discovery of the electrons and protons of the atom came the realization that it is the number and arrangement of these units that determine the particular character of the atom. Matter can be seen as a structure of energy units revolving with immense velocities in space and time. Smuts drew several conclusions: matter is intensely active rather than inert and passive; radioactivity in matter renders fluid the old fixed forms; the structural character of matter indicates that it is creative via its inner activities and forces; and particles dispersed throughout cellular substance show properties necessary for the functions of life. These conclusions began to bridge the gap between matter and life.

Smuts next considered the cell as the second fundamental structure, after the atom, in the basic character of the universe. He discussed the cell's complex structure and functions, most particularly those of metabolism and reproduction. The cell differs from the atom in its greater complexity of structure and function, in the specialization of its parts, and in the system of cooperation among the parts which makes them function for the whole. In the synthesis of functions, Smuts saw clearly that something more than just the parts was in operation; the parts responded to a central pressure. From this consideration of organic coordination and regulation, he elaborated the concept of holism.

The following work is comprised of abridged summary sections from chapters in *Holism and Evolution* (beginning with Chapter Five), reprinted with permission of the estate of Jan Christiaan Smuts.

◎ THE GENERAL CONCEPT OF HOLISM

The close approach to each other of the concepts of matter, life, and mind, and their partial overflow of each other's domain, raises the further question whether back of them there is not a fundamental principle of which they are the progressive outcome. That is the central problem of this work.

Two conceptions of genesis or development have prevailed. The one regards all reality as given in form and substance at the beginning, either actually or implicitly, and the subsequent history as merely the unfolding, explication, *evolutio*, of this implicit content. This view puts creation in the past and makes it predetermine the whole future; all fresh initiative, novelty or creativeness is consequently banned from a universe so created or evolved. The other view posits a minimum of the given at the beginning and makes the process of Evolution creative of reality. Evolution in this view is really creative and not merely explicative of what was given before; it involves the creative rise not only of new forms or groupings but even of new materials in the process of Evolution. This is the view of Evolution today commonly held, and it marks a revolution in thought. It releases the present and the future from the bondage of the past and makes freedom an inherent character of the universe.

Creative Evolution involves both general principles or tendencies and concrete forms or structures; philosophy studies the former, while science has more exclusively concentrated on the latter. Yet both are necessary to reality, and any universal formula of Evolution must include both the general activity or tendency and the concrete particular structure, as one cannot be deduced from the other. ... Both matter and life consist of unit structures whose ordered grouping produces natural wholes which we call bodies or organisms. This character of "wholeness" meets us everywhere and points to something fundamental in the universe. Holism (from ὅλος = whole) is the term here coined for this fundamental factor operative towards the creation of wholes in the universe. Its character is both general and specific or concrete, and it satisfies our double requirement for a natural evolutionary starting point.

Wholes are not mere artificial constructions of thought; they point to something real in the universe, and Holism is a real operative factor, a *vera causa*. There is behind Evolution no mere vague creative impulse or *Elan vital* but something quite definite and specific in its operation and thus productive of the real concrete character of cosmic Evolution.

The idea of wholes and wholeness should therefore not be confined to the biological domain; it covers both inorganic substances and the highest manifestations of the human spirit. Taking a plant or an animal as a type of a whole, we notice the fundamental holistic character as a unity of parts which is so close and intense as to be more than the sum of its parts; which not only gives a particular conformation or structure to the parts but so relates and determines them in their synthesis that their functions are altered; the synthesis affects and determines the parts so that they function towards the "whole;" and the whole and the parts therefore reciprocally influence and determine each other and appear more or less to merge their individual characters: the whole is in the parts and the parts are in the whole, and this synthesis of whole and parts is reflected in the holistic character of the functions of the parts as well as of the whole.

There is a progressive grading of this holistic synthesis in Nature so that we pass from (a) mere physical mixtures, where the structure is almost negligible, and the parts largely preserve their separate characters and activities or functions; to (b) chemical compounds, where the structure is more synthetic and the activities and functions of the parts are strongly influenced by the new structure and can only with difficulty be traced to the individual parts; and, again, to (c) organisms, where a still more intense synthesis of elements has been effected, which impresses the parts or organs far more intimately with a unified character, and a system of central control, regulation and co-ordination of all the parts and organs arises; and from organism, again on to (d) Minds or psychical organs, where the Central Control acquires consciousness and a freedom and creative power of the most far-reaching character; and finally to (e) Personality, which is the highest, most evolved whole among the structures of the universe and becomes a new orientative, originative center of reality. All through this progressive series, the character of wholeness deepens; Holism is not only creative but self-creative, and its final structures are far more holistic than its initial structures. Natural wholes are always composed of parts; in fact the whole is not something additional to the parts but is just the parts in their synthesis, which may be physico-chemical or organic or psychical or personal. As Holism is a process of creative synthesis, the resulting wholes are not static but dynamic, evolutionary, creative. Hence Evolution has an ever-deepening inward spiritual holistic character, and the wholes of Evolution and the evolutionary process itself can only be understood in reference to this fundamental character of wholeness. This is a universe of whole-making. The explanation of Nature can therefore not be purely mechanical, and the mechanistic concept of Nature has its place and justification only in the wider setting of Holism. In its organic application, in particular, the "whole" will be found a much more useful term in science than "life" and will render the prevailing mechanistic interpretation largely unnecessary.

A natural whole has its "field," and the concept of fields will be found most important in this connection also. Just as a "thing" is really a synthesized "event" in the system of Relativity, so an organism is really a unified, synthesized section of history, which includes not only its present but much of its past and even its future. An organism can only be explained by reference to its past and its future as well as its present; the central structure is not sufficient and literally has not enough in it to go round in the way of explanation; the conception of the field therefore becomes necessary and will be found fruitful in biology and psychology no less than in physics.

◎ SOME FUNCTIONS AND CATEGORIES OF HOLISM

Avoiding as far as possible philosophical categories and confining ourselves to scientific viewpoints, we shall now try to consider more closely the concept of the whole and the results flowing from it. We have already seen that the concept of the whole means not a general tendency but a type of structure, a scheme or framework, which, however, can only be filled with concrete details by actual experience. A whole is then a synthesis or structure of parts in which the synthesis becomes ever closer so as materially to affect the character of the functions or activities which become correspondingly more unified (or holistic). It is, however, important to realize that the whole is not some *tertium quid* over and above the parts which compose it; it is the parts in their intimate union and the new reactions which result from that union. But in that union the parts themselves are more or less affected and altered towards the type represented by the union so that the whole is evidenced in a change of parts as well as a change of resulting functions.

The whole thus appears as a marked power of regulation and coordination in respect of both the structure and the functioning of the parts. This is probably the most striking feature of organisms—that they involve a balanced correlation of organs and functions. All the various activities of the several parts and organs seem directed to central ends; there is thus co-operation and unified action of the organism as a whole instead of the separate mechanical activities of the parts. The whole thus becomes synonymous with unified (or holistic) action.

This intense synthesis and unification in the action of a whole involves a corresponding transformation of concepts and categories. Thus, while in a mechanical aggregate, each part acts as a separate cause, and the resultant activity is a sum of the component activities; in organic activity or the activity of the whole this separate action or causation disappears in a real synthesis or unity which makes the components unrecognizable in the unified result. Yet even here we must realize that the whole does not act as a separate cause, distinct from its parts, no more than it is itself something additional over and above its parts. Holism is of the parts and acts through the parts—but the parts in their new relation of intimate synthesis which gives them their unified action.

The whole, therefore, completely transforms the concept of Causality. When an external cause acts on a whole, the resultant effect is not merely traceable to the cause but has become transformed in the process. The whole seems to absorb and metabolize the external stimulus and to assimilate it into its own activity; and the resultant response is no longer the passive effect of the stimulus or cause but appears as the activity of the whole. This holistic transformation of causality takes place in all organic stimuli and responses. The cause or stimulus applied does not issue in its own passive effect but in an active response which seems more clearly traceable to the organism or whole itself. In fact the physical category of "cause" undergoes far-reaching change in its application to organisms or wholes generally. The whole appears as the real cause of the response, and not the external stimulus, which seems to play the quite minor role of a mere excitant or condition.

The most important result of the idea of the whole is, however, the appearance of the concept of Creativeness. It is the synthesis involved in the concept of the whole which is the source of creativeness in Nature. Nature is creative; Evolution is creative, just in proportion as it consists of wholes which bring about new structural groupings and syntheses. The whole involves these new structural groupings out of the old materials, and thus arises the "creativeness" of Evolution, as well as the novelty and initiative which we see in organic Nature. The concept of creativeness which flows from that of the whole has the most far-reaching effects in its application to Nature. Once we grasp firmly the fact that Nature and Evolution are really creative, we are out of the bonds of the old crude mechanical ideas, and we enter an altogether new zone of ideas and categories. But the important point for our purpose is that "creativeness" is simply a deduction from the concept of the whole and is characteristic of the order of wholes in the universe. It is wholes and wholes only that are creative. The formula *omne vivum e vivo* could therefore be generalized and applied to wholes generally. This creativeness issues not only in the origin of new organic species but also in the great Values which are the creations of the whole on the spiritual level.

From this it is clear how also the concept of Freedom is rooted in that of the whole, organic or other. For the external causation is absorbed and transformed by the subtle metabolism of the whole into something of itself; otherness becomes selfness; the pressure of the external is transformed into the action of itself. Necessity or external determination is transformed into self-determination or Freedom. And as the series of wholes progresses, the element of Freedom increases in the universe until finally, at the human stage, Freedom takes conscious control of itself and begins to create the free ethical world of the spirit. Holism thus becomes basic to the entire universe of organic progress and free creative advance, to the Values and Ideals which ultimately give life all of worth it has, and to the Freedom which is the condition of all spiritual as well as organic progress.

But Holism is seen not only in the advance—in the changes and variations forever going forward. It is seen just as much in the stability of the great Types. The new always arrives in the bosom of the pre-existing structure and at its prompting and largely in harmony with it. Its novelty is small compared to its essential conservatism. Variation is infinitesimal compared to Heredity. It is this fundamental unity or unitariness and wholeness in organisms and organic Evolution generally which seems to explain their essential stability as well as the regulation and co-ordination of the whole process—its conservative self-control—if one may use a metaphor.

MECHANISM AND HOLISM

The discussion in the last two chapters has disclosed a grading-up of such structures as can in any way be called holistic; beginning with the physico-chemical structures, into which physical and chemical relations enter; passing on to bio-chemical structures or organisms, into which those relations plus something new, usually called life, enter; and culminating in psycho-physical structures, in which all three relations enter, together with the new elements of mind and personality. In this grading-up, the earlier structures are not destroyed but become the basis of later, more evolved synthetic holistic structures; the character of wholeness increases with the series, and the elements of newness, variation, and creativeness become more marked.

Mechanism is a type of structure where the working parts maintain their identity and produce their effects individually so that the activity of the structure is, at least theoretically, the mathematical result of the individual activities of the parts. With the two concepts of Mechanism and Holism before us, we can see how the natural wholes of the universe fall under both concepts. There is a measure of Mechanism everywhere, and there is a measure of Holism everywhere, but the Holism gains on the Mechanism in the course of Evolution; it becomes more and more as Mechanism becomes less and less with the advance. Holism is the more fundamental activity, and we may therefore say that Mechanism is an earlier, cruder form of Holism; the more Holism there is in structures, the less there is of the mechanistic character, until finally in Mind and Personality the mechanistic concept ceases to be of any practical use.

What is the relation between the earlier (mechanistic) and the later (holistic) elements in composite structures, such as bio-chemical and psycho-physical wholes? How can the material and the immaterial influence or act on each other? This is still one of the great unsolved problems of philosophy, and science finds it no less embarrassing. The tendency for science has as a rule been to look upon the earlier physico-chemical structures as dominant and upon the later holistic elements of life and mind as essentially unreal or as having only an apparent reality. Science looks upon the physical realm as a closed system dependent only on physical laws, which leave no opening anywhere for the active intervention of non-material entities like life and mind. On this view, the activity and causality of life and mind are therefore at bottom essentially illusory. On the other hand, if we have to be guided by our clear and unequivocal experience and consciousness, nothing can be more certain than that our human volition issues in active movements and external actions. Besides, if life and mind were merely ineffective illusions, how could they have arisen and grown in the struggle of existence? While science denies reality to life and mind, the other side retorts by erecting them into vital and mental forces with a substantiality of their own. Thus arises the counter-hypothesis of Vitalism. Both views as a matter of fact are one-sided and misleading; the mechanistic view by ignoring the essentially holistic element in organic or psychical wholes; the vitalistic view by misconceiving the vital or psychic element in such wholes. The fundamental mistake is the severance of essential elements in a whole and their hypostasis into independent interacting entities or substances. Thus body and mind wrongly come to be considered as two separate interacting substances.

In reply to mechanistic Science, it can be shown that the holistic factors of life and mind do not interfere with the closed physical system and that a proper understanding of the laws of Thermodynamics permits of the immanent activity of a factor of Selectiveness and self-direction, such as life or mind, without any derogation from those laws.

Again, in reply to the Vitalists, who invent Entelechy or some other substantive entity for the system of life and mind, it can be shown that no such *deus ex machina* is necessary; that the fundamental concept of Holism suffices to explain the creative, directive, controlling activity of organic and psychic wholes; and that the attributes of life and mind are inherent in the concept of wholes and in organisms and humans as wholes. We thus get rid of the notion of separate interacting entities and view organisms and humans as wholes, which involve both the earlier mechanistic and the later holistic phases of Holism. As we have seen Mechanism to be but an earlier, cruder phase of Holism, the problem essentially disappears. A thorough grasp of the concept of wholes and its consistent application to organisms and humans are thus a solvent for the perennial Body-and-Mind problem. We thus envisage the physico-chemical structures of Nature as the beginnings or earlier phases of Holism and "life" as a more developed phase of the same inner activity. Life is not a new agent with the mission of interfering with the structures of matter; it involves no disturbance of the prior structures on which it is based. Holism has advanced only one step further; there is a deeper structure, more selectiveness, more direction, more control. But the new is a creative continuation of the old and not a denial of or going back on it. Holism as an active creative process means the movement of the universe towards ever more and deeper wholeness. This is the essential process, and all organic and psychic activities and relations have to be understood as elements and forms of this process. No explanation is possible which ignores this active creative inner whole at the heart of all organic or psychic structures; in the light of this whole all apparent contradictions disappear.

The fact of Evolution shows that Holism determines the course and the character of the advance. Thus Holism is pulling all the evolving structures faintly but perceptibly in the direction of greater creative synthetic fullness of characters and meanings, in other words, towards more wholeness. The inner trend of the universe, registered in its very constitution, is directed away from the merely mechanical towards the holistic type as its immanent ideal.

◎ MIND AS AN ORGAN OF WHOLES

Mind is, after the atom and the cell, the third great fundamental structure of Holism. It is not itself a real whole but a holistic structure, a holistic organ, especially of Personality which is a real whole.

Psychology treats mind in man and the higher animals as a factor or phenomenon by itself and analyzes it into various modes of activity, such as consciousness, attention, conception, feeling, emotion, and will. In this work, Mind is viewed from a different angle; it is a form of Holism and it is studied as a holistic structure, with a definite relation to other earlier holistic structures. It has, therefore, a much wider setting and performs more fundamental functions in the order of the universe than appears from Psychology.

Mind springs from two roots. In the first place, it is a continuation, on a much higher plane, of the system of organic regulation and co-ordination which characterizes Holism in organisms.

Mind is thus the direct descendant of organic regulation and carries forward the same task. This is the universalizing side of Mind, and it appears in the conceptual-rational or reasoning activity, which co-ordinates and regulates all experience. Its physical basis is the brain and neural system, which is the central system of regulation and co-ordination in the body. It is thus the crowning phase of the regulative, co-ordinative process of Holism.

In the second place, Mind is a development of an "individual" aspect of Holism which already plays a subordinate part in organisms. In man, it pushes to the front as conscious individuality or the Self of the Personality and becomes as conspicuous a feature of developed Holism as regulative co-ordination, if not more so. This intense element of individuality is the principal novelty in the development of Mind, the real revolutionary departure from the prior system of regulative routine, and in Personality it culminates in a new order of wholes for the universe. Mind in its individual aspect is thus the chief means whereby organic Holism has developed into human Personality.

Mind is in some respects as old as life, but life outran it in the race of Evolution. Besides, Mind needed life as a nurse, and its full development has therefore had to wait for that of life. The extraordinary self-regulation of organisms must, therefore, not be put to the credit of Mind, which was essentially a later development of Holism.

Mind is traceable ultimately to inorganic affinities and organic selectivities. The "tension" of a body in disequilibrium gradually became covered with a vague "feeling" of discomfort, which had survival value; instead of remaining a passive state it became active as *ad-*

tension or attention and ultimately consciousness. Interest became appreciable. Simultaneously the active individual side of Mind developed as conation, seeking, experiment; and from this double basis Mind grew with phenomenal rapidity in the earlier species of the genus Homo.

The individual self-conscious conative Mind is rightly stressed by psychology as the Subject of experience, the Self, and ultimately the Personality. In the universal system of order, this individual appears as a disturbing influence, as a rebel against that order. But the rebel fights his way to victory, achieves plasticity and freedom, and is released from the previous regular routine of Holism. Mind thus through its power of experience and knowledge comes to master its own conditions of life, to secure freedom, and to control the regulative system into which it has been born. Freedom, plasticity, creativeness become the keynotes of the new order of Mind.

This is, however, only one side of mental evolution. *Pari passu* with this individual development the universalizing conceptual-rational side of Mind also develops rapidly; its regulative Reason makes Mind a part of the universal order, and the individual and universal aspects of Mind mutually enrich and fructify each other and, on the level of human Personality, result in the creation of a new ideal world of spiritual freedom. This union of the "individual" subjective Mind with the universal or rational Mind is possible because the individual Mind has itself arisen in the holistic regulative bosom. Pure individualism is a misleading abstraction; the individual becomes conscious of himself only in society and from knowing others like himself; his very capacity for conceptual experience results mostly from the use of the social instrument of language. The individual springs from universal Holism, and all his experience and knowledge ultimately tend towards the character of regulative order and universality. Thus knowledge assumes in the first instance the form of an empirical order, as a system of common sense. Gradually, the discrepancies of this system are eliminated, and knowledge approximates to science, to a scientific conceptual order, in which concepts and principles beyond empirical experience are assumed to underlie the world of experience. The scientific world-conception marks the triumph of the universal element in Mind but only on the basis of the freedom and control which the individual mind has mainly achieved. Mind as an organ of the whole, while taking its place in the universal order, has emancipated itself from the earlier routine of regulation and has assumed creative control of its own conditions of life and development. Thus it creates its own environment in society, language, tradition, writing, literature, etc., instead of being dependent on an alien environment as on the organic level. Again, Mind frees itself from the intolerable burden of organic inheritance by inheriting merely the widest, most plastic capacity to learn and letting the social environment and tradition carry on the onerous duty of recording the past. While the animal is hidebound with its own hereditary characters, the human Personality is free to acquire a vast experience in his individual life.

Mind has its conscious illuminated area and its subconscious "field." In this field, the forgotten experience of the individual life as well as the physiological and racial inheritance exercises a powerful influence. It is this influence that proves decisive for our fundamental bias, our temperament, our point of view, and our individual outlook on persons and things. It is of an intensely holistic unanalyzable character; it is even possible that our neural endowment carries with it more in the way of sensation and intuition than appears from the special senses; that the sensitive basis from which they have been differentiated has continued to develop *pari passu* with them and today forms a subtle holistic sense, a capacity of psychical sensing or intellectual intuition which explains our holistic sense of reality as well as other obscure phenomena, such as telepathy. So much for the influence of the past. The future also becomes a potent influence on Mind. Through its dual activity of conception and conation, Mind forms "purposes" which envisage future situations in experience and make the future an operative factor in the present. Purpose marks the liberation of Mind from the domination of circumstances and indicates its free creative activity, away from the trammels of the present and the past. Through purpose, Mind finally escapes from the house of bondage into the free realm of its own sovereignty. All through its great adventure, its procedure is fundamentally holistic, and this can be shown by reference to the various activities of Mind as analyzed by psychology. Free creative synthesis appears everywhere in mental functioning and not least in the region of Metaphysics, Ethics, Art, and Religion, which, however, fall outside the scope of this work.

◎ PERSONALITY AS A WHOLE

Personality is the latest and supreme whole which has arisen in the holistic series of Evolution. It is a new structure built on the prior structures of matter, life, and mind. The tendency has been to look upon it as a unique and isolated phenomenon, without any genetic relations with the rest of the universe. Our treatment, however, shows it to be one of a series, to be the culminating phase of the great holistic movement in the universe.

Mind is its most important and conspicuous constituent. But the body is also very important and gives the intimate flavor of humanity to Personality. The view which degrades the body as unworthy of the Soul or Spirit is unnatural and owes its origin to morbid religious sentiments. Science has come to the rescue of the body and thereby rendered magnificent service to human welfare. The ideal Personality only arises where Mind irradiates Body and Body nourishes Mind, and the two are one in their mutual transfigurement.

The difficult question of the Body-and-Mind relation . . . arises once more in connection with Personality. . . . the root of the difficulty lies in the separation of the elements of Body and Mind and their hypostasis into independent entities. They are not independent reals; disembodied Mind and disminded Body are both impossible concepts, as either has meaning and function only in relation to the other. The popular view of their relation as one of mutual "interaction" is not correct, as Mind does not so much act on Body as penetrate it and thus act through or inside it. "Peraction" or "intro-action" would be preferable to "interaction" as a description of the relation of Mind to Body. The extreme difficulty of conceiving how two such disparate entities as Mind and Body can influence each other has led to various theories of their inter-relation, such as—that God is the medium and agent between them . . . ; that their separate action is inwardly brought into accord by a Pre-established Harmony . . . ; that they are but two modes of action of the one underlying Substance. . . . The fact is that all these theories have an element of truth; the real explanation being that Mind and Body are elements in the whole of Personality and that this whole is an inner creative, recreative, and transformative activity, which accounts for all that happens in Personality as between its component elements. No explanation will hold water which ignores the most important factor of all in the situation, and that is the holistic Personality itself. Holism is the real creative agent. . . .

We see this same creative Holism in Personality when we come to consider our inheritance from our parents and ancestors, which consists of a definite animal body slightly differing from theirs and a mental structure somewhat resembling theirs. My Personality itself, however, is indisputably mine and is not inherited from them. It may in some respects resemble theirs, but its very essence is its unique individuality. The fact here too is that Personality is a unique creative novelty in every human being and that no explanation which ignores this creative Holism can even pretend to account for Personality.

◎ SOME FUNCTIONS AND IDEALS OF PERSONALITY

The central conception of Personality is that of a whole; it is the most holistic entity in the universe; hence no other category will do justice to it, and certainly not mechanism. Psychology is too much of an abstract science to give an adequate view of Personality, though even psychology is dependent on the theory of a central synthetic activity for the correct construction and interpretation of mental experience and ignores that theory at its peril. The suggestion of a new science or discipline of Personology has therefore been made which will study Personality more synthetically and concretely than is possible for psychology.

As an active living whole, Personality is fundamentally an organ of self-realization; the object of a whole is more wholeness, in other words, more of its creative self, more self-realization. This means that the will or active voluntary nature of Personality is its predominant element, and the intelligence or rational activity is subordinate and instrumental—it has to discover and co-ordinate means to the end of self-realization. Feeling is likewise subordinate, its function being to give strength and impetus to the will. The Personality is thus a more or less balanced whole or structure of various tendencies and activities maintained in progressive harmony by the holistic unity of the Personality itself. In fact, Personality resembles an organized society or state with its central executive and legislative authority wielding sway over its individual members in the interest of the whole. Kant has rightly called man a legislative being. Part of this control in Personality is conscious; most of it is, however, subconscious. This control is still largely imperfect and immature owing to the extreme youth of Personality in the history of Evolution. But it is growing. More holistic control in the Personality means greater strength of mind and character; better co-ordination of all impulses and tendencies; less internal friction and wear and tear in the soul; more peace of mind; and finally that spiritual purity, integrity, and wholeness which is the ideal of Personality. The Personality has the same self-healing power which we saw already in the case of a mutilated organism, and in case of moral or other aberration it usually has the power to right and recover itself and often creatively to gather strength from its own weakness or errors.

Personality is not only a self-restorer; it is a supreme spiritual metabolizer; it absorbs for its growth a vast variety of experience which it creatively transmutes and assimilates for its own spiritual nourishment. As metabolism and assimilation are fundamental functions of all organic wholes, the Personality takes in and assimilates all the social and other influences which surround it and makes them all contribute towards its holistic self-realization. Personalities vary greatly in their capacity for holistic assimilation, some easily suffering from spiritual indigestion, while great minds and characters can absorb a vast experience which only serves to fructify and enrich them without any detriment to their spiritual wholeness and integrity. Where a Personality takes in alien experience which it cannot assimilate into its own spiritual substance, such experience becomes an impurity to it; "purity" in reference to Personality meaning the absence of all elements alien, heterogeneous, and disharmonious to the Personality. . . .

The essence of Personality is creative freedom in respect of its own conditions of experience and development; as an initiator, metabolizer, and assimilator it has practical self-determination. Again, as a selector and co-ordinator of the elements in the situations that confront it, it also has practical freedom. Its very nature as a whole confers freedom upon it. This freedom is not a negation of the physical order of causality but arises inside that order; holistic freedom is a continuous organic or psychic miracle which happens *between* cause and effect. . . . Freedom is thus a fact in the universe and is not a mere capricious power peculiar to the will; it pertains to Personality as a whole. Freedom means holistic self-determination, and as such it becomes one of the great ideals of Personality, whose self-realization is dependent on its inner holistic freedom.

As regards Wholeness or Purity, it is essentially identical with Freedom. Purity means the elimination of disharmonious elements from the Personality. It means the harmonious co-ordination of the higher and lower elements in human nature, the sublimation of the lower into the higher, and thus the enrichment of the higher through the lower. From this, it follows that moral discipline is an essential part in the culture of Personality. Personality is a spiritual gymnast, whose object is the freedom and harmony of the inner life through the refinement and sublimation of the cruder features in the Personality and their subordination and co-ordination in the growing whole of Personality. If this object is secured by the Personality, all the rest will be added unto it: peace, joy, blessedness, goodness, and all the great prizes of life. Wholeness as free and harmonious self-realization thus sums up the *summum bonum* of Holism.

THE HOLISTIC UNIVERSE

The fundamental, seminal character of the concept of Holism is bound to affect our general views of the nature of the universe, our *Weltanschauung*, and this chapter deals with this wider aspect of Holism.

Holism has been presented in the foregoing chapters as the ultimate synthetic, ordering, organizing, regulative activity in the universe which accounts for all the structural groupings and syntheses in it, from the atom and the physico-chemical structures, through the cell and organisms, through Mind in animals, to Personality in man. The all-pervading and ever-increasing character of synthetic unity or wholeness in these structures leads to the concept of Holism as the fundamental activity underlying and co-ordinating all others and to the view of the universe as a Holistic Universe.

On a strict and narrow view, Science may consider the concept of Holism as extra-scientific, as giving a metaphysical and not a scientific explanation of things. But this would be a mistake for three reasons. In the first place, the conclusion to which Science is pointing, namely, that the whole universe, inorganic as well as organic, is the expression of cosmic Evolution, necessitates a ground-plan which will formulate and explain this vast scientific scheme of things. Mere pre-occupation with detailed mechanisms will no longer suit the immensely enlarged scope of present-day Science. In the second place, Science has already had to assume such ultra-scientific entities as, for instance, the ether of space, as necessary to give a coherent explanation even of purely physical phenomena. And the correlation of the physical, and organic, and psychical in one vast scheme of Evolution similarly necessitates much more widely operative factors than have been hitherto recognized. Holism is far more necessary for cosmic Evolution than was the ether for light transmission. In the third place, Holism is essentially no more ultra-scientific than are life and mind; it is simply a wider concept than either and is the genus of which they are the species. And it enables all the evolutionary phenomena of Nature to be co-ordinated under and traced to the same operative factor.

The New Physics has traced the physical universe to Action, and Relativity has led to the concept of Space-Time as the medium for this Action. Space-Time means structure in the widest sense, and thus the universe as we know it starts as structural Action; Action which is, however, not confined to its structures but continually overflows into their "fields" and becomes the basis for the active dynamic Evolution which creatively shapes the universe. The "creativeness" of evolutionary Holism and its procedure by way of small increments or instalments of "creation" are its most fundamental characters, from which all the particular forms and characteristics of the universe flow.

The ignorance or neglect of these two fundamental characters accounts for the elements of error involved in certain widely held world-conceptions, such as Naturalism, Idealism, Monadism, and Spiritual Pluralism or Panpsychism. Naturalism is wrong where it fails to recognize that there is creative Evolution and that real new entities have arisen in the universe, in addition to the physical conditions of the beginning. Idealism is wrong where it fails to recognize that the Spirit of Psyche, although now a real factor, did not exist either explicitly or implicitly at the beginning and has arisen creatively in the course of organic Evolution. The Monadism of Leibniz and his modern sympathizers, while a great advance in that it recognizes the inward holistic element in things and persons, yet goes wrong when it attributes an element of Mind or Spirit to physical things like atoms or chemical structures. While things are wholes they are not yet souls, and the view of the universe as a Society of Spirits ignores the fact that spirit is a more recent creative arrival in the universe and cannot be retrospectively antedated to the earlier material phase. Spiritual Pluralism is a modern refinement of Monadism and similarly subject to the criticism that it fails to recognize the really creative character of Evolution.

This is a universe of whole-making, not of soul-making merely. The view of the universe as purely spiritual, as transparent to the Spirit, fails to account for its dark opaque character ethically and rationally; for its accidental and contributory features, its elements of error, sin, and suffering, which will not be conjured away by an essentially poetic world-view. Holism explains both the realism and the idealism at the heart of things and is therefore a more accurate description of reality than any of these more or less partial and one-sided world-views.

Nature or the Universe is sometimes metaphorically spoken of as a Whole or The Whole. Sometimes it is even personified, and the trend of Evolution then becomes the Purpose of some transcendent Mind. All this is, however, unwarranted by the facts and unnecessary as an explanation of Evolution. Holism as an inner evolving principle of direction and control in all Evolution is enough; it underlies the variations which arise and survive in the right direction, and it creates in the "field" of Nature a general environment of internal and external control. The "wholeness" or holistic character of Nature appears mostly in this field or environment of Nature, with its friendly intimate influences, and its subtle appeal to all the wholes in Nature, and especially to the spiritual in us. The fact is that the Holism in Nature is very close to us and a real support in all our striving towards betterment. Our aspiration is its inspiration, and it is thus the inner guarantee of eventual victory in spite of all set-backs and defeats.

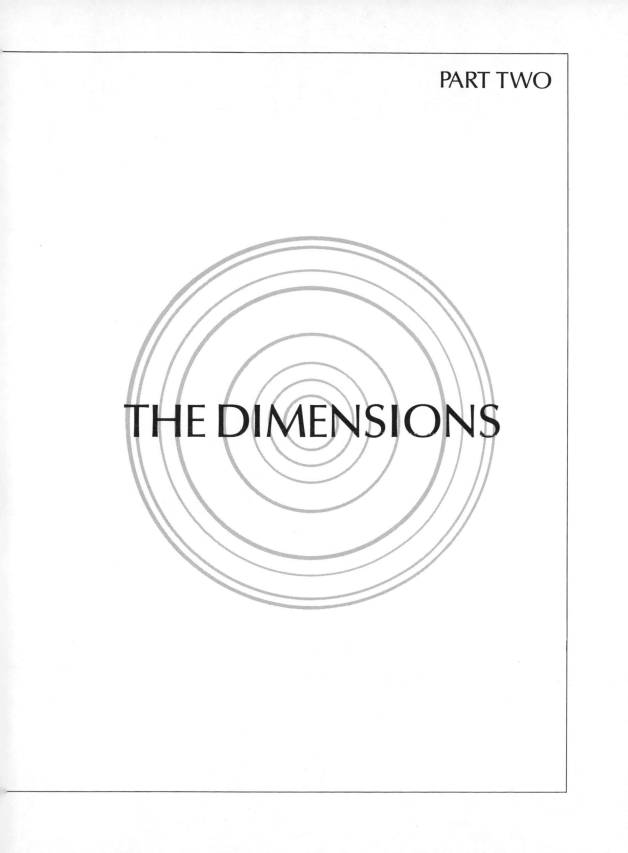

PART TWO

THE DIMENSIONS

2

THE NUTRITIONAL DIMENSION

RUDOLPH BALLENTINE, M.D.

The variables that affect the nutritive value of what we eat are complex indeed. Vitamin, mineral, and protein content vary not only from food to food but also from foods grown in one area to those grown in another. The value of the protein, for example, also depends on the way in which various foods are combined, and the amount of carbohydrate we need depends on our activity and way of life. Moreover, each person's needs vary according to his individual makeup, his personality, and his way of reacting to situations around him, so some people have higher requirements for one vitamin and lower requirements for another. The amount of food assimilated from that which is taken in depends to a great extent on the functioning of the digestive system. This varies from person to person, but it may also vary from day to day or even hour to hour, depending on our emotional or mental state. We may secrete more enzymes or less, depending on our state of mind and on our attitude toward the food, what it might mean to us, or whether it looks and tastes appealing. Climatic and seasonal variables also enter into the picture and have an effect on our requirements.

If we all vary in our psychological makeup and, because of this, use our bodies in different ways so that our nutritional requirements vary, how then do we go about finding out which diet is a good one for us? Faced with the complexity of choices in diet, with biochemical individuality, and with the unpredictability of daily needs, it becomes quite apparent that we cannot calculate mathematically what our requirements are.

Clearly, the optimal selection of food is a matter that defies our intellectual capacity. No amount of education and training prepares us to consider all these multiple variables in ourselves and in the food before us. We must therefore rely on taste, appetite, instincts, feelings, impulses, and intuition. After we have learned to recognize what is wholesome and what is not, we must then make, from the best available foods, a selection that is based on our inner promptings. Despite all the elaborate information that is available on the biochemistry of nutrition, the cues provided by our own system are the most reliable guide.

Somewhere in the conflicting impulses and urges that arise into our awareness when we think of eating are the data that we need to guide us to the food that our bodies require. These internal indicators have to be patiently trained. What is often referred to as hunger, for example, is not really hunger at all but rather the socially or psychologically conditioned urge to eat. We have to filter out all other connections involved with food, tuning in to the correct signals and tuning out the static. This is not always easy, but as we learn from experience which signals are reliable and which aren't, we gradually gain facility in distinguishing those which will not mislead us, and these signals become clearer and easier to perceive. The result is a cooperative effort between our mind and body which provides the information needed to select the food that is most appropriate at a given time.

In our struggle to cope with old habits, to increase our sensitivity to ourselves, and to open our eyes to ways in which we have misused our digestive system and body, we will learn much. Not only will we learn about nutrition, we will also gain important insights into the emotional and physiological aspects of our nature. It has long been known that many of our deepest psychological problems and most serious emotional conflicts show up most clearly in our dietary habits. Such frank abuse is often covered up by the most amazing blindness. It is not uncommon to have a patient who has undergone some treatment with training in nutrition and dietary awareness remark, "I never realized what I was doing to myself!"

Learning to deal with food and what it means to ourselves becomes, then, an *autopsychotherapeutic* process. Mixed in with those signals and cues that reflect a true need for certain nutrients are many other impulses and associations which have to do with our past. The sight or smell or taste of a certain dish may bring back memories or associations of a pleasant experience or of someone who was loved and with whom a certain food was shared. Sometimes these memories may not come fully into awareness, and we may feel an inexplicable urge to eat something for which our body has no use at the time. Food may symbolize many things, which gives it attraction quite apart from its nutritional value. Eating certain food with another person may be a way of feeling closer, while eating other food may provide a stimulation or mask an allergy.

From the ancient Eastern perspective, consciousness is potentially much more capable of influencing the way the body functions and the way it handles food than is the food itself. Yet it is curious that, while the Eastern point of view relegates diet to an inferior place in the scheme of variables affecting the human being, it is in the East where diet is managed in the most sane and healthful fashion. The Westerner, whose philosophy would suggest that his material being is of utmost importance and that, moreover, "he is what he eats," tends to constantly violate all the rules that he has acknowledged lead to good health. Even from an Eastern perspective, it is a serious waste of time to chase after organic produce and count milligrams of vitamins to the point that we become harried and flustered and require more of the nutrients we're trying to get! Though food may be less important than our state of mind in determining the overall nutritional picture, it still plays a role.

Though the mind affects nutrition in numerous and complex ways, what was eaten today can also affect our present clarity of consciousness. As we struggle to become more aware of ourselves and of what food does to us, our diet itself may, at the same time, be one of the most potent means of assistance we have. It has been found, for example, that both human infants and laboratory animals, when allowed to select freely what they will eat, chose more wisely and did much better if they had been well nourished up to the time that they were put on their own.[1] Those who had been on a poor diet for some time seemed confused and unable to select the foods they needed. Good nutrition fosters the development of "body wisdom," we might say—just as sensitivity to body cues fosters good nutrition.

As we shall see, what we can learn intellectually about the rational selection of food and the deliberate design of diet is probably inferior to a highly developed intuitive sense of what we need. Yet it may be precisely that contrived diet and schedule which bring enough regularity and sanity to our eating habits to clear our heads and enable us to begin to reawaken and cultivate our innate sense of what is appropriate and right for us.

Sorting out the signals and becoming aware of our non-nutritional reasons for eating results in more than simply getting a good diet. It is really a process of self-study, a continuing adventure in self-exploration, a progressive untangling of past memories and conflicts, and a way of coming to terms with them. Working out and overcoming our cravings often involves working out and overcoming deep-seated psychological conflicts. This work with the food, the schedule, and the eating, then, is the battleground on which such conflicts may be resolved. Their resolution in terms of food may, in many cases, amount to their psychological resolution. Thus, this process of working through can be therapeutic in a total sense rather than being merely an improvement in diet.

Only those who have struggled sincerely with their eating habits can appreciate the profundity of this concept. It is said in the East that, "he who would attain enlightenment must first conquer the palate." Diet, like any other area of our lives, if approached in the right spirit, can become a means to growth and personal fulfillment. For this reason, a quiet, persistent approach to diet involving self-study and a cultivation of increased self-awareness might properly be called "food *sadhana*." "Sadhana" is a Sanskrit word meaning "pathway" and is often used to denote that particular practice by means of which one works toward personal fulfillment and spiritual evolution.

Once we begin to approach the subject of nutrition from a personal, experiential point of view, new horizons open. For instance, if we make a careful study of the effects of different foods on ourselves, we will begin to find that we can classify them into different categories. What's more, we will begin to learn interesting things about ourselves—our feelings, our desires, our conflicts. In the East, there are many systems that provide the framework within which we can do this, such as the Ayurvedic system.

Developing our fullest capacity for studying ourselves in relationship to our food calls on the best of contemporary scientific data on nutrition and physiology combined with the essence of ancient traditions of organizing the experiential data of self-observation. But the rewards are worthwhile, both in terms of improved nutrition and in personal growth.

MAKING OURSELVES INTO NUTRITIONAL LABORATORIES

Studying nutrition from an experiential approach requires that we prepare ourselves. If the outcome of an experiment is to be clear and intelligible, it must be carried out where conditions are stable and predictable. The laboratory must be in good order. We can't do productive research in the midst of confusion and chaos. The setting must be quiet, calm, and constant. In other words, a laboratory is a place where we can keep constant most things that would affect an experiment, focusing on only one. This one is then changed so that the results can be studied. Whatever happens must have been due to the change that was made, since everything else remained the same.

In working with the body and diet, if our system is functioning smoothly, it becomes a suitable laboratory. After eating something different, if the body reacts strangely, or the mind becomes fuzzy, it is possible to have some idea of what caused it.

There are several steps that are preliminary to beginning to discover the proper foods. These steps clear the field so that our experiments are not obscured. The first is to adjust the quantity of food eaten. If a lot of food is piled into the system, the system is going to be clogged. It is possible to overwhelm the capacity for the digestion of food. The enzymes are limited in amount, and they can only handle so much. The Charak says, "One must eat in proper measure and the proper measure of food is determined by the strength of one's gastric fire,"[2] and in a later verse, "The self-controlled man always feeds his gastric fire with the fuel of wholesome food and drink, mindful of the consideration of measure and time."[3] If too much is put in, it piles up, bacteria begin to grow in it, and the result is wastes and contaminants that mess up the internal laboratory. Trying to learn about diet in such a situation would be like trying to work in a lab where huge boxes of supplies were piled, where perishable things had spoiled, and where containers were knocked over and their contents spilled so that everywhere one turned there was another collection of garbage. In the midst of all that, it would be impossible to isolate one variable and study it successfully.

So the first order of business is to be sensible about the *quantity of food* eaten—to provide a cleaner body in which to work. If a reasonable amount of food is put into the body, a lot of digestive problems disappear, and the system begins to function in a quieter, less confused way.

The next matter of importance is *when we eat*. It is often necessary at first to get on a fairly regular schedule, eating at set intervals. If we skip two out of three meals on one day and then eat six times on the next, our system will often be upset, regardless of whether we are eating the particular food our body needs or not.

Scheduling should be such that there is more or less the same pattern each day. For most people, two meals a day are enough. If you feel more comfortable with three, then the schedule should include three. But to have four or five or six feedings a day is almost always unnecessary (even in those who are susceptible to hypoglycemic episodes). If the digestive tract is full of food and, before it even begins to be processed and digested, more is dumped in, how can we know what is the effect of what? It becomes difficult if not impossible to know whether the feelings we experience are due to the juice we drank at eight o'clock, the granola and bananas we had at nine, or the "mid-morning snack" at eleven.

If, on the contrary, we eat one meal and then wait five hours or six hours before eating another meal, the digestive system has time to finish what it is doing before it starts over. This is important not only to facilitate self-study but also because the "machine" doesn't work well otherwise. It's not designed to have a constant input. Whenever something is put in the mouth, digestive juices are secreted, and a definite series of processes is triggered. If we have breakfast at eight o'clock in the morning, for example, the whole system is set into motion. Food goes through the intestines, juices are secreted in each place, and digestion is completed. Once the process is over, there is a "clean-up," after which the digestive tract is ready for another dose of food. That may be at one or two o'clock in the afternoon.

Therefore, the first and most obvious step toward establishing the conditions that will enable us to learn more about the effects of food is to apply these commonsense principles to the use of the digestive system. Once these simple matters are in order, we can begin to discover which specific foods are best for us. It is only necessary to eat the food in question and to observe the results. If the effects of the experiment are not immediately obvious, then it may be necessary to take the food once or twice a day for several days to see the changes it makes. Is there more gas? Does the stomach always feel full? Is there a feeling of heaviness and fatigue? Is the mind sluggish? These are, of course, indications that what was eaten doesn't agree. An excess of mucus is another indication, as is a bad taste in the morning or offensive breath.

Dietary changes should be made gradually. Becoming vegetarian on Tuesday after having a half a chicken on Sunday and a jumbo sirloin on Monday is not helpful. Drastic changes will yield no useful information. They may produce reactions—sometimes dramatic ones—but this usually provides little understanding. Overzealous and self-righteous "reforms" in diet are ill-advised.

In the Charak Samhita it is written:

> By degrees the wise man should free himself of unwholesome habits; also, by degrees he should develop wholesome ones. The acquisition of the new good habits and the giving up of the old bad ones should be achieved by regular quarter-steps of decrease at orderly intervals of one, two and three days.[4]

This allows us to settle gradually into a new eating pattern. Not only is this approach more likely to establish lasting changes, it provides more opportunity for observation. It is said that Gandhi changed his diet regularly to learn how it affected him. That is true, but he changed it only every four months. Thus, he was able to conduct meaningful experiments. Though our research on ourselves may not allow us to draw statistically supported conclusions, it does open new realms of self-awareness.

If living habits are reasonable, regular, and sane, we will begin to notice that we have certain impulses or feelings that a particular food is either not suitable or is "just what we need." Such a subjective sense of what is right can be a valuable guide. Even experimental animals distinguish between a mixture containing all the essential amino acids and an otherwise identical mixture which lacks one of them. Horses will choose the feed with the most minerals, and cows will graze bare a strip of pasture grown organically leaving the chemically fertilized grass standing around it.[5] In the case of man, this intuitive sense of what is best, or what is needed at the moment, can be sharpened and refined.

Diet and Self-Regulation

As we begin to tune in to inner cues, we encounter a variety of urgings and impulses. Some are based on habit and past conditioning, while others are based more on current and realistic needs. To sift and sort through these requires a lack of distraction, ample time, and a process of retraining ourselves. If we have lost touch with these inner cues and are trying to re-establish contact and awareness, we will find conversation, noise, a tight schedule, and other distractions a great hindrance at first. In the Ayurvedic scriptures, where experiential awareness of diet played a central part, certain suggestions were laid down for the practice of eating:

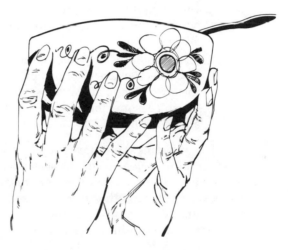

Figure 2–1.   Diet and self-regulation.

1. *Eat alone.* At the beginning of re-educating ourselves and our attitudes toward food, it is often helpful to be alone during meals. This allows time to pay attention to the taste of the food, its texture, and the way it affects our bodies. It allows time to tune in and consult the body, asking, "Do I need more? Have I had enough? Do I need some of this or some of that?"

2. *Chew carefully.* The Ayurvedic scriptures suggest chewing each bite 32 times, "once for each tooth." Prolonged chewing makes us more aware of the food we are eating. It also allows us to digest it properly. The taste of food varies during the full process of chewing. The full spectrum of tastes that occurs

during the proper chewing of a bite of food allows the body to assess its properties and develop a feeling about what such food supplies, how much more is needed and so forth.

3. *Choose an appropriate amount*. It is helpful to serve the amount which we think is appropriate, to go off alone, eat it, and then be finished. This removes the tendency to overeat or undereat and allows us to learn to gauge how much we need. Another approach is to eat only one food at a time, chewing thoroughly and pausing between bites, eating that food until we have had enough and then going on to what seems to be appealing next. If this is done thoughtfully and with full attention, if only wholesome foods are offered, and if foods are selected according to what seems to be needed rather than what might taste interesting, then surprisingly enough, we do not overeat. In fact, this approach has been successfully used for weight loss.[6]

4. *Select appropriate foods*. Other, more complex, guidelines to food selection are provided by the Ayurvedic principles, which specify which foods could be expected to be appropriate during which seasons, for which sort of people, at what time of day, and so forth.

The guidelines that have been laid down for helping a person who is attempting to learn how to select his food properly are not to be followed slavishly in a mechanical or rigid way. No one can determine what is right for another person to eat. Although a nutritionist may make general statements about what the average person needs, he may have more trouble determining exactly what is right for himself.

In the ancient cultures of the East, people were trained in self-observation, and rules for sane living were regarded as valuable aids in establishing the conditions that permitted experimentation. Inner experimentation became a way of life. To the modern urban dweller, who keeps strange hours, eats a hodgepodge of processed and semi-artificial foods, and rushes around in his polluted environment, the ancient Indian would appear regimented and unimaginative. The truth may be different.

Regularity of living was valued not as an escape from variety and change but rather as providing the freedom to experience it. In India, rules are generally followed but widely regarded as made to be broken. A self-regulatory approach to diet requires constant experimentation and exploration. The proof of the pudding is in the eating. Sometimes what is right is what seems to be most contrary to all the rules.

The story is told of an Irishman, lying on his deathbed, who was asked by his physician whether he had a last wish. Rallying enough to reply, the dying man responded, "Yes, I would like a cold pork pie and a bottle of stout." His wife shuddered, sure that it would kill him, but the doctor took her aside and gently reminded her that, since her husband could not, in any case, recover, it would be best to let him have this last wish fulfilled. So a friend was dispatched to the corner pub and soon returned with the pie and stout. The patient swallowed it down almost in one gulp, whereupon he stood up looking much improved. He then proceeded to make a rapid recovery.

The rules are not hard and fast. There are times when they should be broken—if for no other reason than to simply see what happens when they are. They are not really rules at all, in the usual sense of the word, but guidelines to help in establishing conditions that will facilitate inner experimentation.

Learning to be aware of our real needs and taking in what will satisfy them is not the easiest of challenges to meet. Habits often lead us to eat when we're not hungry or to eat things for which our bodies have no use. There are many signals and urges we will experience. Some are based on taste appeal and associations with past experiences. Others are based on genuine physiological needs. To sift and sort through these requires much attention, thoughtfulness, and sensitivity. A Spartan approach and an attitude of self-denial is of no help. To the extent that we can tune in to our physiological cues and select our food appropriately, we will feel clearer, more alert, and more comfortable and content. What we know about the biochemistry of nutrition (vitamins, minerals, fats, carbohydrate, protein) and of digestive physiology, combined with what we have learned of more traditional ideas about nutrition and our perception of our internal signals, leads, upon each encounter with food or appetite, to a hypothesis: "I think I need *this*, and it will probably make me feel *that* way." Then we are ready to proceed with the experiment (eating) so we can collect the data (see what happens). But it is the internal cue that gives the whole experiment meaning, since this cue ties the meaning to subjective experience in a way that allows us to gradually sharpen and come to trust our urges and impulses.

When properly trained, appetite, tastes, and bodily cues can be very accurate and dependable sources of information about what we need nutritionally. Moreover, they change from moment to moment and keep us current as to what is needed and what is not. If we're emotionally upset, we lose our appetites. This is the way our physiology has of advising us that digestion would be difficult at this time. Unfortunately, these cues are not always acknowledged or recognized.

Too often, the small, still voice of our inner urgings is overwhelmed by the noise around us, the force of our habits, the pressure of peer groups, and the curiosity to try foods for which we have no real appetite. Too often, we eat according to our schedules and according to what is convenient rather than according to our needs.

There is a story told in the East of two fakirs who had spent years in seclusion studying yoga, having learned extraordinary feats of physical and mental control and mastery of their minds and bodies. They encountered each other on the banks of the Ganges, and, in the course of their conversation, one of them happened to imply that he had developed the ability to do more miraculous things than most, probably including his companion.

The other fakir, a bit older and perhaps a bit wiser, rebuked him gently, wondering whether he might not be carried away by a moment's boastfulness. But his newfound friend bristled with pride and volunteered to demonstrate what he could do.

The older man agreed to this. "Go ahead," he said.

The younger proceeded, "See the man across the river? I will make appear on a piece of paper in his hand the name of a friend whom he has long forgotten."

The older man smiled, "Is that really the sort of thing you do? That's nothing."

The younger fakir replied, now with some heat, "Oh, really! That's nothing? Well, please tell me, what sort of miraculous feats do you accomplish?"

The first fakir looked at him calmly, and his eyes twinkled, "I eat when I'm hungry and drink when I'm thirsty."

If one can eat only when hungry and yet, at the same time, take his meals with reasonable regularity and at proper intervals, he will have met one of the greatest challenges of good nutrition.

From what has been said, it should be clear that the schools of nutrition that have grown up in ancient civilizations are based more on experiential data than experimental data. By that is meant that the understanding of what is appropriate food for each person is based more on the information that each person has at his immediate disposal—his feelings, his sensations, his ideas, and his sense of himself—not on the kind of particularistic, mechanistic, molecular analysis that must be carried out in a specially equipped laboratory. This is partially true, of course, because the technology required for this latter kind of external, material study was not available in the older civilizations. In any event, interest was focused more on the interface between man and food: a field of data that can best be apprehended by an inward turning of attention, an experiential self-observation of internal events that precede, accompany, and follow the intake of food.

INTERACTION BETWEEN NUTRITION AND THE MIND: A SPIRAL

As a part of the process of sharpening our awareness of internal events, it is helpful to consider the effects that the mind may have on our nutritional habits. The interactions between mind and diet can form distinct patterns, notably downward or upward spirals.

As the mind becomes disturbed, a person loses touch with the subtle signals that cue him to what is appropriate to eat and when. If, for example, he becomes more irritable and emotionally disturbed, his eating habits are very likely to become more erratic. Not only may he fail to take meals on time, skipping some entirely, but out of nervousness, restlessness, or simply a lack of awareness, he may overeat or eat too often. Poor dietary regulation leads to poor intake of nutrients and deficiencies, which, in turn, makes us more irritable and mentally and emotionally disturbed. The result sounds like the classical "vicious circle."

Unfortunately, this cycle is not merely circular. A circular process would show no net change for better or worse. Actually, however, there is often a gradual but definite worsening—a sort of building crescendo of emotion, unbalance, and erratic living habits with poor dietary practices. The result, instead of a circle, is a downward-moving spiral.

Effects on the Liver and Other Organs

The interaction beteen the diet and the mind may involve, as an intermediary step, effects on the liver. The liver plays an important intermediary role in maintaining an internal homeostasis and balance. All the nutrients coming from the intestinal tract (with the exception of a large proportion of the fats) go to the liver, where they are processed before they are released in the bloodstream. The liver is also responsible for filtering the blood and removing any wastes, contaminants, or toxins that might damage the cells throughout the body or interfere with their function. The liver serves to provide a constant internal milieu in which the nervous system can function, and if it does its job properly, it contributes greatly to our ability to maintain a sense of equanimity, calm, and peace of mind.

If the liver is not functioning properly, many of these toxic materials remain in the blood and are circulated throughout the body. This can cause an overall heaviness, achiness, and soreness, as well as an unmodulated supply of nutrients. These circulating wastes, metabolites, and contaminants are, in some cases, able to enter the nervous system and may directly interfere with the functioning of the brain and central nervous system. This can create feelings of apathy, lethargy, and often depression.

First and foremost in the therapeutic approach is the proper regulation of the diet, since the liver is forced to cope with whatever is absorbed by the intestinal tract and brought to it by the portal vein. It is clear, then, that the liver is a strategic link between nutrition and the mind, serving as an intermediary through which they interact in many ways. When the digestive fire (or *pitta*, in the Ayurvedic tradition) is properly regulated, energy is said to flow evenly and consistently from the solar plexus, giving a feeling of vitality and well-being. When this fails, however, accessory organs of regulation that should normally be pushed into extra activity only in an emergency situation must take over.

Other organs may also serve as strategic links that mediate the primary interaction between the diet and the mind. The pancreas is often involved. It may put out too much, too little, or poorly timed insulin, and it may do the same thing with glucagon, the hormone that releases stored glucose. Its production of digestive enzymes can also be affected so that the tense, usually angry, person who suffers from hypoglycemic spells may also have difficulty with digestion and absorption.

The stomach is also prone to be caught up in the spiral of interaction between diet and mind. Certain personality traits and attitudes toward the world, such as suppressed hunger and dependency and a tendency to turn angry feelings inward, may be reflected physiologically by increased gastric acid and the "eating away" of the stomach's lining.[7] This often leads to overeating or snacking to keep the stomach full. When the extra foods are sweets, they may trigger a further secretion of acid.[8] On the other hand, hopelessness, depression, and feelings of inadequacy may be related to an inadequate secretion of gastric acid,[9] which weakens protein digestion and drops the protective barrier against bacterial overgrowth in the small intestine, culminating in flatulence, indigestion, and again, an overloaded liver—the sum total of which clearly accentuates feelings of depression and inadequacy and completes one more turn of the downward spiral.

Fortunately, such downward-moving spirals as that occurring with disordered sugar metabolism can move in the other direction, too. If we become more alert and aware of the physical symptoms that guide the proper intake of nutrients and regulate our diets according-ly, we will often find that our nervousness diminishes, our mental state improves, and we are able to think more clearly. This, in turn, allows us even finer and more successful regulation of our eating hab-its, which, in turn, again improves our nutrition and diminishes our nervousness further. In other words, the cycle need not be vicious. It can move in a quite beneficial direction, toward balance. But when the spiral moves further and further away from balance and homeo-stasis, its downward course may carry us toward any number of chronic, degenerative, and pathological conditions. The direction that we take may hinge on many factors besides physiological makeup, which is actually, to a great extent, dependent upon other variables, such as the symbolic meaning that food holds for us and our past hab-its and experiences that have resulted in self-destructive tendencies and attitudes of which we may be only partially aware.

Obesity as a Downward-Moving Spiral

Another example of a downward-moving spiral is obesity. The kind of discomfort and craving that results from the overall lack of nutrients often seen in overweight people, especially when they are dieting, is quite different from what a healthier person calls hunger. Obese peo-ple, in fact, seem relatively insensitive to hunger. If no food is taken for some time, contractions of the stomach and reductions in blood sugar take place that would be interpreted by most people as hunger. In experimental situations, obese subjects, however, reported no feel-ing of hunger at that time.[10, 11] On the other hand, when snack foods were available, overweight persons who had just eaten a full meal ate more than a similar group with empty stomachs.[12]

Apparently, people who tend to become overweight are insensi-tive to the inner cues that should let them know when food is needed and when it is not. Learning to tune in to internal states is, then, an essential feature of any successful program for losing weight.

Though people who are overweight tend to ignore the internal signals that should regulate eating, they often respond to external signals. Besides being habituated to eating when food is present, they may respond to emotional situations by stuffing themselves with food. When put in a situation that aroused fear, a group of overweight persons did not "lose their appetites" as did those of normal weight. In fact, they ate more.[13] If we are to lose weight and keep it off, we must be involved in some systematic effort to learn new ways of handling

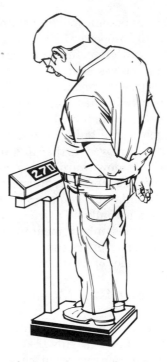

Figure 2–2.   Obesity, a downward-moving spiral.

stress and emotional upset. Methods of relaxation, breathing, bio-feedback, or meditation not only provide successful techniques for this purpose but also promote the kind of body awareness that the obese person so badly needs to learn.[14]

Exercise fits this bill, too. Not only does it help in diverting attention from food-oriented matters, it also, obviously, burns up calories. In one study of a group of teenage girls, those who were overweight ate no more than their classmates, but they were much less active.[15] It has been estimated that a secretary who exchanges her manual typewriter for an electric one, but keeps her diet and living habits otherwise the same, will gain four to six pounds a year. Without increasing the general level of physical activity, it is impossible for most people to lose weight. To maintain the reduction, it will be necessary to make physical activity a more prominent part of their lifestyle, even after weight is lost.

Regularity is part of this. If meals are erratic and unplanned, then scheduled exercise never comes off. Either a person is about to eat and is not in the mood, or he has just eaten and can't exercise with a full stomach. For those who are seriously overweight and have lost touch with their inner cues, a regular schedule of meals is almost a necessity. If the diet is also rich in non-caloric nutrients that regularly satisfy genuine needs, it may be possible to gradually re-establish enough order in the internal chaos so that healthy and meaningful appetite signals can be perceived.

If carefully followed, a regular schedule of meals also does much to cut through an obsession with food. If we know, "Now I eat. Now it is over; nothing else until next meal," then the constant internal dialogue about whether to eat or whether to practice self-restraint can be eliminated. This frees a great deal of energy which can be invested in other activities that gradually provide new fulfillment and open new horizons.

Weight loss must be the by-product of personal evolution. The person who tackles the weight problem head on, as though *it* is the basic issue, is doomed to fail. If a person does not truly outgrow being fat, he will lose (and gain) tons in a long and unhappy career of dieting struggles.[16]

It must be remembered, too, that weight loss is a process of "uncovering." What emerges from the layers of fat during this process is not only a new, thinner person but also the problems and conflicts that led to overeating. If a person is prepared to come to terms with such issues as how he has closed the door on inner signals and feelings, how the tendency to be inactive relates to habits of thinking and feeling, and what the self-image of "fat" means to him, he will become less burdened psychologically as well as physically.

Cultivation of body awareness, learning techniques for handling emotional distress, and finding new avenues for self-fulfillment and creativity, along with establishing habits of physical activity and maintaining a balanced, simple, sensible diet especially rich in vitamins, minerals, and high-quality protein, can be successful. Such a program does not mechanistically or automatically remove weight from a fat person, but it does provide the conditions under which a fat person can sometimes "outgrow being fat."

Food Allergy and Food Addiction

Apparently, some people have extremely strong reactions to certain substances in natural foods. Such a reaction is called a "food allergy," and some of then have been dramatic. Researchers in this area report full-blown psychotic episodes, for example, emerging almost instantly as a drop of an extract of the food to which the person is sensitive is placed under the tongue.

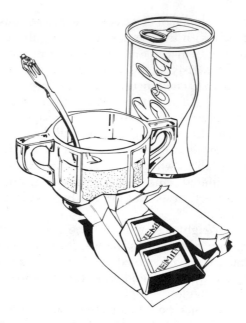

Figure 2–3. Food allergy and food addiction.

Allergic reactions are not always so dramatic. They may constitute only a mild feeling of unease, flushing, a runny nose, a headache, or any number of other miscellaneous aches and pains that seem to appear for no apparent reason. You need not go through the drama of having the food put through a stomach tube to test for food allergies. You can just as easily test yourself at home by taking your pulse after eating some food suspected of causing trouble. If the pulse is markedly elevated,[17] then you know you are sensitive to the food in question.

Physicians who have studied such problems call themselves *clinical ecologists*. By identifying which foods cause the reaction, they are able to eliminate them. On careful testing, however, a patient is seldom found to be allergic to only one food.[18] Problems are commonly caused by such foods as wheat, corn, eggs, and milk. To eliminate several of these from the diet, however, is not practical for most people. In children, this can be especially true, since, by avoiding many of the available nutritious foods, they can miss important nutrients and become seriously malnourished. Fortunately, by eating small quantities of a food that causes some reaction, a person can usually build up a tolerance for it, whereas taking large amounts alone can aggravate the condition. Moreover, the substances in food to which we become allergic are proteins, and cooking often denatures such proteins so that they lose their power to trigger allergic reactions. Thus, a person sensitive to raw milk or even pasteurized milk may suffer no ill effects from milk that is boiled.

Even pinning down exactly which foods are the culprits may not be so easy. Immediate reactions can be picked up by sublingual tests, but the delayed reactions that are thought to occur days later are very difficult to identify. We may be mistaking a delayed reaction to a food taken yesterday for an immediate reaction to something just eaten. Sometimes a total fast is carried out for several days to a week or more. Then foods are gradually added, one at a time, to observe their effects.

The approach of clinical ecology is to look at other factors in the environment besides food that might cause trouble. Dust and mold are often offenders, and to eliminate them may require special carpets, draperies, etc. Though some persons find themselves allergic to one discrete substance and by simply eliminating it obtain some relief, it is usually a combination of things that must be avoided. The whole program can become very complicated and awkward:

Mrs. G saw a well-known clinical ecologist for a stuffy nose. As a test for allergies, she was fasted and then given large amounts of the food suspected of causing trouble. On the day she ate six scrambled eggs, she felt very ill. Similar reactions resulted from other foods such as wheat and milk products. She was counseled to avoid all these foods and to be careful to use only organically grown produce. Finding the foods she could eat became quite difficult. This was especially true since she was found to react adversely to exhaust fumes and so couldn't drive an automobile. She would spend her day on the phone locating usable items, and her husband would go in his time off work to purchase them. He began to tire of this and to suspect that she did it to provoke him. The situation between them was worsened when, because of pollens and dust, they were advised to move to a different town. Though he gave in, foods continued to upset her, and the doctor insisted that anything which caused any negative reaction should be avoided. Since by now almost any food seemed to cause her to feel giddy or sluggish, she ate very little. She lost weight, her skin became discolored, and she developed strange and uncontrollable cravings. On one occasion, she ate one-and-a-half pounds of honey at a sitting and felt "a great sense of relief and well-being." At this point, a glucose tolerance test showed hypoglycemia, so she put herself on a high-protein diet, but that made her feel dull. She tried the climate in the Southwest, but the water in the hotel was chlorinated, which gave her a bad reaction. After one frightening weekend when she couldn't get anyone to bring her water by automobile, she fled, terrified, feeling herself a fugitive from the world.

The allergist calls this perspective "exogenous," i.e., the cause of illness or distress is seen as external to the person.[19] This means, of course, that correction of the problem requires alterations in the environment and in the food supply rather than in the person himself. Not only is this cumbersome and unwieldy, it does little to help the patient outgrow and overcome his problems. It may be more useful to adopt a different viewpoint and ask what it is internally that sets the stage for such a reaction.

Food Allergies and the Mind

Allergic reactions are a result of malfunctioning of the immunologic system. The immunologic system is one of the body's first lines of defense. It manufactures antibodies to combat "foreign" materials—those that "don't belong" in the body. The antibodies attach to the foreign materials and help in their destruction and elimination from the body. In this way, the body rids itself of bacteria and viruses, as well as many other useless and potentially harmful protein substances. Occasionally, however, things go haywire. The body "recognizes as foreign" a protein molecule that is actually customarily present in the digestive tract. Why this happens is not known. Recent research suggests, however, that it may stem from an unhealthy digestive tract—one where the usual barrier to foreign proteins is compromised. In the healthy bowel, the wall of the intestine serves as a sort of sieve. It allows small molecules, such as amino acids, through but not larger ones. Antibodies are made only of peptides—strings of amino acids. So when the intestinal wall is healthy, food allergies should be unlikely.

Moreover, recent research has begun to turn up some interesting information about the control of immune responses. In experimental animals, when certain small areas of the brain are destroyed, antibody production is affected.[20] Significantly, it is precisely those areas that are most closely involved with emotional states where tissue destruction disrupts immune responses. This particular point in the brain, called the *hypothalamus*, is both part of the "circuit" that is active when one is anxious or upset and a bridge to the pituitary gland, which regulates the secretion of hormones. Certain hormones are thought to play a role in the regulation of antibody production, too, and it is thought that mental and emotional states affect the way a person reacts to a foreign substance by means of this complicated network.[21] This is probably particularly true in the case of those reactions we call "allergic."[22]

If future research bears this out, we may find that the "diagnosis" of food allergy and the attention and anxiety it arouses in the patient may actually do more to aggravate the situation than it does to help it. Certainly, in most cases, it is true that a balanced, healthful diet of wholesome foods, along with a well-designed program of relaxation, breathing exercises, and other techniques to improve the ability to handle stressful situations, will enable most persons with "food allergies" to eventually overcome them.

Behind the allergy usually lies a complex of problems and difficulties of a psychological nature. To invest energy in a continual quest for everchanging "permissible" foods and in a constant struggle to avoid dust, animals, or pollens, is an attempt to escape the work that we are faced with and to retreat into an uncomfortable status quo.

◎ THE HOLISTIC PRACTITIONER'S APPROACH

Our Combined Therapy Program at the Himalayan International Institute in Honesdale, Pennsylvania, is designed to apply holistic principles. To this end, we combine several therapies in order to address all aspects of the person. We may use physical therapy and exercise, meditation, yoga, homeopathy, allopathic medicine, herbal medicine, Ayurvedic medicine, psychological counseling, and nutritional counseling.

Though nutrition is one way to approach the problems a person brings to the practitioner, there are alternate ways of helping people besides changing their diet, and there are other things besides diet that are important to consider. If an individual does ask for a diet, then we say, "Come in and let's evaluate you first and get to know you, and then we will give you whatever guidance we believe is appropriate for you. If diet is the tool you want to work with, then let's work with it." If the person should find that he is better able to work with himself from another point of view, then diet will come along later in our work.

The first thing we do is work toward understanding the whole person. We do a full physical examination, take the person's medical history, and do a psychological examination. The physical exam may include conventional laboratory tests as they are indicated. The medical history includes information about any kind of illness that the person has had in the past; a complete family history, including whatever problems his parents and grandparents suffered from; and any kind of symptoms that the person is having currently. The psychological exam gives an understanding of how the person functions psychologically; yet it does not assess his mental status in any mechanical sense.

In addition to going through the person's medical records, we must get to know the person, his habits, his occupation, and the way he lives his life. It is necessary to have a comprehensive assessment of the individual; in fact, it is impossible to do nutritional counseling from a holistic point of view unless the practitioner understands the whole person. Otherwise, it is a farce and is neither holistic nor nutritionally sound.

Reaching this understanding of the individual takes at least an hour or two—at times, it is not until the second or third visit that an overall understanding is reached. Each time, we look at the person's diet record and find out what he eats.

Rather than ask questions to do a nutritional assessment, we have the person bring a record of everything he has eaten for the last four days. A practitioner usually cannot discover what someone really eats by asking him what his diet is because a person's retrospective recall of what he eats is often distorted. He may try to impress the practitioner with how conscientious he is about his diet, he may actually forget certain items he felt guilty about when he ate them, or he may unintentionally leave out certain things that he is embarrassed to mention.

The four-day record is accurate for the most part. Certainly, a record is more objective than an oral description. If the person genuinely wants help, he will conscientiously write down everything that he is eating. This, in itself, he usually finds revealing. "I had no *idea* what I put in my body in the course of a day," is a common remark. The therapeutic work, the cultivation of self-awareness, has already begun before the person walks into our office. After studying the four-day diet record, we explain which foods may have adverse effects on the person's health. Then we make recommendations as to which foods can be eliminated and which should be added, how these foods should be prepared, and in what combinations they should be eaten. Usually, we work toward a simple basic diet of whole foods: grains, beans, vegetables, a little fruit, maybe a little milk, and some supplementary foods.

As the person notes how the changes affect his health, revisions are made to refine the therapeutic goals of his diet. A diet is developed with the person over a period of time, and any dietary advice is tailored to the unique needs of the individual.

Diagnosis

It has been said that it is just as difficult to change a person's eating habits as it is to change his character structure. Actually, the two are essentially the same. There are always definite relationships between a person and his eating habits, and these relationships need to be understood in the holistic diagnosis. People with certain kinds of health problems will tend towards certain eating habits as a general rule. This does not mean that people with the same problems will eat exactly the same foods, but they will approach diet in certain ways: they will tend to eat a particular kind of food, overdo in one area, or eat on specific kinds of schedules, and so forth.

The relationships between certain character structures and their tendencies can be very subtle, so they cannot be directly classified in the way that personality types are classified in psychiatry. It is possible, though, to look at a person and guess what he does with his diet or to be given his diet and have a rough idea of what the person would be like.

We can make correlations, further, by using a combination of thinking in terms, for example, of <u>Ayurvedic diagnosi</u>s and tridosia, homeopathic remedies, certain aspects of degenerative disease that result from overusing one kind of food or another, and other ideas that come from practical experience and are more difficult to describe.

Perhaps the clearest example of this kind of correlation is in homeopathy. It is definitely true that given homeopathic remedies fit given character structures; that certain character structures will need certain remedies. It is possible to observe a person walking, to watch how he sits and how he talks, and then to guess the homeopathic remedy that is appropriate for him. The case of a young woman I met on a plane provides an illustration.

In conversation, this woman mentioned that she had certain medical problems. From the way she talked, the way she was built, and her whole constitution and personality, I knew what homeopathic remedy she would need. Then I could predict what other symptoms she probably had—for example, problems with her fingernails breaking and problems with her menstrual periods occurring too often and lasting too long. Because I knew what the remedy was, I knew what additional symptoms went with that remedy and what the prominent symptoms would be. Of course, when I mentioned these other symptoms to her, she was somewhat taken aback! So, there's a definite correlation between personality type and homeopathic remedies. Homeopathy utilizes substances that come out of nature, and the nature of the substance is reflected in the nature of the person whom it will help.

If an individual has a certain constitution and has symptoms or certain kinds of disorders, this is often associated with certain kinds of dietary habits. These habits then show up in his bodily make-up, so an experienced practitioner can estimate what the person's diet is like and what his health condition is like.

In terms of diet, there are people who eat too much; who eat too often; who eat large quantities of fats and oils; who consume a lot of sugar; who like hot foods, spicy foods, heavy foods, or bland foods; who eat a lot of milk and eggs; and who absolutely cannot stand any fat meat or any kind of fat yet crave butter. There are people who won't eat any kind of fat and people who eat all fats. There are all these different varieties and more.

Certain attitudes and medical problems are correlated with these dietary patterns. Some dietary habits and patterns do correlate with a wide number of symptoms in many different physical and mental subsystems, and some of these patterns are recurring. An individual, for example, who hates fat or the fat part of meat is often the person who has cancer or will get cancer. The same may be true of the person who craves fat—either extreme indicates an imbalance. There is the person who craves carbohydrates and gets fat, and the one who craves carbohydrates and doesn't get fat. Often, the one who craves carbohydrates, eats eggs, and gets fat is very frightened and has sweaty hands.

A classic example of such a pattern is the person who craves sugar, is hypoglycemic, and has pancreatic problems, a bad temper, hypersensitivity, and keloids (large and visible overgrowths of scar tissue). This person may be preoccupied with sex, react intensely to sounds like the scraping of fingernails on a blackboard, and frequently get sties in his eyes. These are all overreactions that indicate an imbalance.

Another example of a pattern is the person who eats a lot of protein, especially meat. He tends to be overheated; has a high body temperature; is restless, impatient, easily angered, and sweats a lot; has kidney problems; and has bags under his eyes. This person tends to come down with diseases like gout, arthritis, and heart disease.

Because each person is so distinctively different, though, we can really only make these correlations and diagnoses while working with the person. At this point in the diagnosis, we can begin to develop a strategy for treatment, can see what are the most important things to change first, and can establish priorities.

Treatment

Out of everything we have examined about a person, we should now have some sense of the most important thing that the person is doing wrong. What is the thing that's hurting him most or standing most in the way of his health or his awareness?

There can be one, two, or several obstacles which we rank in importance. If a person has severe arthritis, for example, we may attend to the sugar or meat in his diet. If it's someone with heart disease, we might be more interested in the fat of the diet. Another factor that we must consider, based upon what we know about the person, is what changes we expect he will most readily accept. We may change only two or three things initially and give the person time to notice the effects of these changes on his health before we look at him again. We may use other therapies, such as homeopathic remedies, Ayurvedic remedies, or whatever else is appropriate, along with that diet so that the diet is not prescribed separately from the other things. The effects of the remedies (to catalyze psychophysiological change) and of other interventions (such as psychotherapeutic strategies, biofeedback, etc.) that also contribute to personality and physiological reorganization all act to shake things loose so that the person is ready to experiment with new dietary patterns and new attitudes toward food.

Essentially, when the whole person has been evaluated, we evolve a plan that may include diet, remedies, exercise, certain concentration exercises, breathing techniques, etc. Then when the person comes back, the same thing happens again: we sit with him, look at him, listen to him, feel his presence, and assess him. Then we determine what things would help his growth at this point. It may be more clear at this stage in what direction this person seems to be trying to move, how it is that he gets hung up and is not moving, and what would help him in terms of his growth in that direction. Another plan should emerge from this evaluation; a plan in terms of diet, remedies, and so forth.

These things are synergistic. The diet without the other things will not do very much. Working together, the diet and the exercise program, remedies, meditation techniques, and whatever else is included in the plan, are all more powerful.

It is especially important to span the whole spectrum of levels on which the human being functions and attend to each of them. No area should be completely overlooked. If there is one area where growth is most important or where the person is trying to work, then this area should be supported. If the right area is being focused upon, then other areas of the person do come along. This is always true. Each person functions on physical, emotional, mental, spiritual, and energy levels. The person may be amenable to work in one area above others in terms of his interests, his capabilities, his past experiences, and what he's prepared to work with. If he works effectively in that area—maybe it's through breathing or some way of developing his awareness of energy, for example—then certainly, this work is going to help his physical health, his psychological health, and his spiritual health. If improvement on other levels isn't seen, then the therapy should be re-evaluated. Usually, two or three levels can be worked on at the same time, if the person is sincerely involved and interested.

We tell participants in our program that they must come for a minimum of two weeks; they must be motivated; they must pay in advance; and they must commit themselves to this. We work with people on several levels. We help each individual evolve a diet. We bring the person's food to his room so that he eats alone and learns to pay attention to the food, to chew the food, and to sense the food. We ask him to go in the kitchen, watch the cooking, learn to prepare the food, and then to hear six hours of lectures on nutrition in order to understand more about diet.

Food is only one part of the program. The same thing applies to exercise. If the person is the right age, we do a treadmill EKG, evaluate his exercise capacity, help him design an exercise program, and work with him in terms of stretching exercises, aerobic exercises, hatha yoga, and whatever else he can do and develop at home by himself.

We also work with breathing. We do breathing tests in various situations to see how the person's breath responds, and we help him analyze his breathing habits and develop practices to improve them. Breath is considered especially important since it is thought to directly affect the energy patterns operative in the psychophysiological complex.

A similar approach is used with meditation. We teach the person how to evolve a systematic way of studying and understanding his thought processes, not in the dyad or in the group, but on his own, so he can do it constantly, and it can become part of his way of existing. Self-observation then becomes part of his nature; it doesn't stop. If he develops it in meditation, it becomes part of the way he lives. There we see one of the many interlinkings that make the various modalities of a holistic program work synergistically: the cultivation of introspection and self-awareness will markedly enhance the work with diet. The critical cues that effective self-regulation in nutrition must depend on are internal cues. Unless we learn to be increasingly aware of the inner world, dietary changes will be merely mechanical. And when that's true, we drop them very soon. Of course, the analysis of the thought processes also leads to psychological reorganization. So, in our program, the person has hours of lecture on meditation and how to analyze the mind introspectively through a technique that comes from yoga.

We also look at posture and teach the person how to be aware of it and how to work with it. The same level of intensity is applied in all aspects of what we do. We are working intensively while, at the same time, helping people learn about the therapeutic tools (so they can go further with them after they leave) and giving the remedies that catalyze changes and bring data into awareness. Once the remedies have brought things into awareness, the person has something to work with using the techniques that we've been talking about. With all these levels working together simultaneously, the results are fantastic.

The process involves a long period of time because people don't change overnight. In our program, the process is initiated; it isn't finished. This is why it's as much a training program as a treatment program. Rather than trying to cure a disease, we are approaching the person as a whole human being and trying to help him move on his way to wherever he's going. The physician is his consultant, who offers him some guidance on things he can do with his diet and exercise program and so forth that will help him on his way. Once he finishes the two weeks at the Himalayan Institute, if he finds that he's making progress and doesn't need any consultation, we may not hear from him for a year or maybe never again.

Whether in the live-in (Combined Therapy) program, or in one of our outpatient clinics, the goal is for the person to learn to take care of himself. After a certain point, say, two, three, or four visits, most people start to catch on to what to look for and what to do; that's the whole point. People need not traipse around after doctors for the rest of their lives. Individuals can learn as much as they want to.

In Honesdale, we offer courses in the use of homeopathic remedies at home, we sell kits, and we teach people how to manage minor things themselves. If they don't have any major constitutional problems or degenerative diseases or anything serious, then why should people need to see a doctor? There are Ayurvedic guidelines for what to eat and what herbs and spices (which are really medicines) to use. Anyone who has studied yoga and meditation in depth begins to get a sense of Ayurveda.

Certainly, it is possible for people to learn these things; though they're not learned intellectually, they are learned experientially. The more a person works in consultation with one of the physicians in our clinics, the more he begins to get a sense of how to assume that perspective and stance, and the more he is able to do it for himself. So we say that our patients graduate from treatment, and they don't come in any more. They know what to do. They get a little out of balance, they sense it, understand it, and know how to correct it. They don't have to come in and ask what to do. It is our purpose to educate people—to have them learn how to take care of themselves and make their own discoveries. In this way, they can go off and grow in their own direction.

Once a person gets a sense of how that's done, he no longer has to run to a doctor every time he discovers something. It is a much more effective approach than telling the individual what he should do and handing him the "correct diet" to follow. The authoritarian position of the doctor accomplishes very little, and that only on a short-term basis.

The goal, then, of any successful nutritional approach is for a person to become more sensitive to himself, more aware of the choices that he has, and more attuned to how the consequences affect him. Self-awareness must be allowed to grow. Experience with food must become part of an ongoing experiment in an inner laboratory. In this way, nutrition study takes its place alongside such other methods of self-examination and inner searching as the various forms of psychotherapy and meditation.

By getting in touch with the cues that a person's body offers him, the individual can decide what is appropriate to eat and what is not. Through sharpening his awareness of himself and his reactions to foods over a period of time, a person can evolve dietary habits and practices that seem comfortable, natural, and conducive to health. The use of this approach to nutrition lends flexibility and the capability for constant change. The individual no longer needs to establish a plateau of nutritional status. He need not settle into a rut. Instead, he is free to go through a process of evolution. As his body and mind change and evolve, he is also able to reorganize his dietary habits so that, at each stage of transition, they shift to meet his new needs, continually creating states of greater health and alertness.

REFERENCES

1. R. Williams, *Physician's Handbook of Nutritional Science* (Springfield, IL: Charles C Thomas, 1975), pp.95-96.

2. *Charaka Samhita*, Sutrasthana 5:3, Vol. II, p. 68 (Jamnagar, India: Shree Gulabkunverba Ayurvedic Society, 1949).

3. *Charaka*, Sutrasthana 27:345, Vol. II, p. 557.

4. *Charaka*, Sutrasthana 7:36-37, Vol. II, pp. 114-115.

5. L. Alther, "Organic Farming on Trial," *Natural History* 81 (1972): 230.

6. C. Gerrard, *One Bowl* (New York: Random House, 1974).

7. H. Davenport, *Physiology of the Digestive Tract* (Chicago, IL: Year Book Medical Publication, 1977), p. 184.

8. T. Cleave, *The Saccharine Disease* (New Canaan, CT: Keats Publishing, 1975), p.147.

9. Davenport, *op. cit.*, p. 184.

10. A. Stunkard, "Obesity and the Denial of Hunger," *Psychosomatic Medicine* 21 (1959): 281-289.

11. A. Stunkard and C. Koch, "The Interpretation of Gastric Motility," *Arch Gen Psychiat* 11 (1964): 74-81.

12. S. Schachter, "Obesity and Eating," *Science* 161 (1968): 751.

13. *Ibid.*

14. T. Thorpe, "Effects of Hatha Yoga and Meditation on Anxiety and Body Image," in *Meditation Therapy*, ed. Swami Ajaya (Glenview, IL: Himalayan Institute, 1977).

15. M. Johnson, B. Burke, and J. Mayer, "Relative Importance of Inactivity and Overeating in the Energy Balance of Obese High School Girls," *Am J Clin Nutr* 4 (1956): 37.

16. Gerrard, *op. cit.*

17. A. Coca, *The Pulse Test* (New York: Lyle Stuart, 1956).

18. S. Klotz, "Allergy Screening Consultation Service to an Inpatient Psychiatric Service," in *Clinical Ecology*, ed. L. Dickey (Springfield, IL: Charles C Thomas, 1976), pp.708-718.

19. T. G. Randolph, "Historical Development of Clinical Ecology," in *Clinical Ecology*, ed. L. Dickey (Springfield, IL: Charles C Thomas, 1976), pp. 9-17.

20. M. Stein, *et al.*, "Influence of Brain and Behavior on the Immune System," *Science* 166 (1969): 435-440.

21. *Ibid.*

22. K. Pelletier, *Mind as Healer, Mind as Slayer* (New York: Delta, 1977), p. 65.

3

THE MOVEMENT DIMENSION

ANNA HALPRIN AND
DARIA HALPRIN-KHALIGHI

Movement is a change of mass from one place to another, and this happens when the bones are shifted by the muscles. In organizing the bony structure, the muscles contract and release. In order to move, there has to be one set of muscles that contracts, another set that releases, and then a rest period. The contraction, release, and rest pattern is a basis for rhythm. Rhythm is a natural attribute we all have.

Developing this idea further, our natural capacity for rhythm involves organization of the elements of space, time, and force. Take, for example, the automatic, naturally occurring phenomenon of breathing. Notice your breathing as you are reading this page. When you inhale, your breath consumes a specific amount of time, occupies space, and is felt with a particular degree of force. As you breathe out, these elements may change. Take a moment and explore ways you can change your breath rhythm—speed up, slow down, hold your breath, make the intervals between breathing in, out, and resting even, then uneven. There are endless combinations. When you are frightened, anxious, or nervous, your breath rhythm will reflect this state by becoming fast and hard. Anger can make your breath rhythm slow and intense. When you are relaxed and calm, your breath rhythm slows down; the interval of exhaling increases, and the degree of force becomes soft and gentle. The next time you experience uncomfortable emotions, such as anxiety, fear, or anger, and you would like to change, try paying attention to your breath—slow down, exhale deeply, take a long rest before inhaling, and see if shortly your uncomfortable feelings will have altered. Within the biology of our bodies, we have the natural capacity to use rhythmic awareness as a useful and an immediately available way to enhance our health and well-being.

Rhythmic movement varies with the state of health. In order to acquire optimal rhythmic movement we need to:

1. move in partnership with gravity,
2. move all the parts of the body as a whole body,
3. move congruently with the intention of the function or task,
4. move with kinesthetic aliveness,
5. move with appropriate expressiveness.

A person moving in an integrated way moves with ease. In a simple movement like swinging the arms in an arc from left to right with

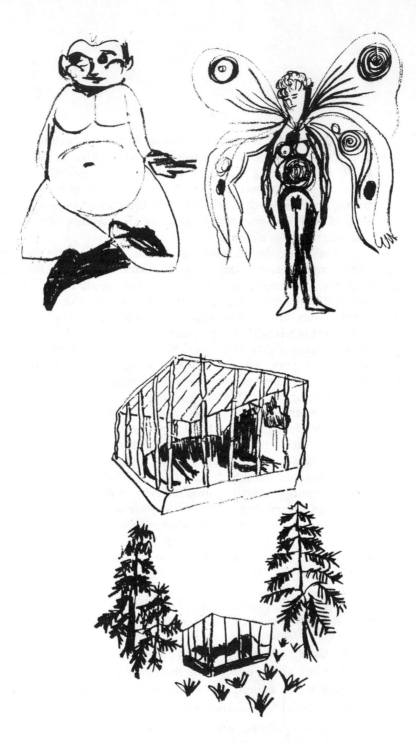

Figure 3–1. Drawings made by dance workshop participants before and after workshop experiences.

the head following, the entire body—knees, torso, neck, everything—is included in the movement. The head follows smoothly, the torso twists slightly, and the knees flex. In healthy movement, the body responds as a whole in accordance with the function of the movement. The breath is full, deep, and effortless, with its rhythmic flow harmonious with the intention of the movement.

Whenever the interaction between the five points mentioned above is out of order, the body is forced to counterbalance in a way that triggers off misalignments throughout the body and its movements. A movement generated from one part of the body will trigger off a set of responses from the whole body mobilizing around the movement.

If any part of the body is out of contact with the whole body, or if any part of the body is not moving through a natural accommodation for the movement, one piece of the body will be rigid or stuck. The breath will, as a result, be shallow and often held in; the stuck part will be creating effort and tension. With continuous misuse, patterns in the body become habitual. Chronic symptoms result, such as joint degeneration, tight muscles, lower back pain, eye strain—any number of common complaints. We can learn to use movement to avoid injury and instead promote health and creativity. For example, if we have developed a habit of holding the breath and not breathing fully, we affect the entire rib cage. Often, we find that not breathing fully causes the rib cage to become tight because the intercostal muscles are stuck. When we are breathing fully and are relaxed, we can put our hands where the intercostal muscles are and feel movement in the rib cage with every inhalation and exhalation.

◎ EMOTION

Another way imbalance affects the whole person is in building physical and emotional tightness. This is especially true of people who tend to work intensely. These people tend to have longer intervals of contraction; more time is spent on the contraction and not enough time on the release of the muscles. For every second that we contract, our muscles may need as much as 10 seconds to release in order to maintain proper rhythmic balance. People under constant pressure do not get enough release. With lack of release and relaxation, tension builds up. Tension will lodge in different places in the body, and where it lodges may depend upon the personality. For a stubborn person, it may lodge behind the neck; for a sexually frightened person, it may lodge around the hips; for a person who restrains from moving and taking action, it may lodge in the thighs and legs. Tension will go to different places in the body which reflect different emotional sets we have.

◎ MOVEMENT

Movement Awareness

When we begin to pay attention to our movements, we are learning *movement awareness*. This awareness can begin when there is feedback between movement and feeling. Movements are connected to feelings through our nervous system. We move all the time for utilitarian purposes, and we never question such movement, whether we are getting dressed, eating, walking to get somewhere, or driving a car. But that is not the only way we move. We also move for non-utilitarian purposes. We move to express how we feel, whether we are aware that we're doing this or not. It is natural to make a gesture, for example, as an emphatic kind of movement when we are expressing a feeling. This kind of movement can mean that we are putting ourselves out to someone or holding ourselves back. We can make a point with a certain brazenness or anger by slamming one fist into the other open hand. But our movement towards a baby will be very gentle. We are constantly moving in relationship to feelings.

Expression and Order

When we connect movement to feelings, with awareness, we immediately begin to initiate *expression*. When our expression is consciously understood—in other words, when we commit ourselves to conveying this expression—we must give the movement expression, order, and organization—that is dance.

Life, in all its forms, is a manifestation of a quickening force sensed as energy. Coexistent with this force, and regulating its flow, is the phenomenon of rhythm. Without its principle of order and proportion all would be chaos. Its presence is revealed in the life patterns and forms of all organic processes. Man/woman and everything he/she does are subject to its rules or organization. Nothing escapes. Feelings and thought, as well as actions, are subject to this rhythmic scheme. Thus, dance, itself an expression of organic and bodily rhythm, must be considered as an extension of emotional and intellectual rhythmic form, projected into and through movement.[1]

Once movement ordering begins, dance may evoke feelings, thoughts, fantasies, associations, and myths which are transforming and transpersonal. The thoroughness or the depth to which we can go into our movement in relationship to our responses, and the extent to which we can order and articulate, will give us the possibility of connecting to a force larger than ourselves. One person's sadness or joy is an expression that others can experience because others have the capacity to feel the same way. That communication is immediately a transforming act: we transform from our individualities to a collective identity. We have gone beyond our own subjective feelings. Whether the feeling is humor, whether it connects with a myth, or whatever particular form it may take, others can *empathize* with us.

From the point of view of health, this is the tremendous value of movement and dance. When we can go through ourselves and become bigger than ourselves, there is a sense of release. Something about the ability to connect with a universal principle or a force larger than ourselves has the effect of causing release. The process takes us out of ourselves and gives us a broader perspective; we see ourselves as part of a universal whole. By including our own personal self into a larger force, it is as if we become part of nature and are once again reaffirming our harmony with nature. This is the connectedness between our nature and the larger nature and the point of release in the harmony of reconnecting to nature through universal principles.

Therapeutic Approaches to Movement

There are many different therapeutic approaches to movement (movement therapies) to help people release tensions and strengthen and balance themselves. Certain of these may be used more for structural reintegration, muscular retraining, biofeedback and diagnosis, and awareness enhancement, and others may be used for coordination and development of vital energy. Feldenkrais, the Alexander method, bioenergetics, Trager, rolfing, polarity, applied kinesiology, yoga, t'ai chi ch'uan, and dance are some techniques used in holistic health.

Individuals may learn any one of these disciplines or therapies and benefit tremendously in developing their movement awareness. We have chosen dance, as we feel it is a natural and creative approach to movement. Our workshops are designed to give people the opportunity to explore their own inner material, move through emotional blockages, and express themselves freely without being limited to a certain form. This is why we teach only the basic principles of movement and dance, not a single style or school of dance. We develop *with* people an understanding of movement awareness that they can use throughout their lives, a process that they can make their own and that allows for continuous growth and creativity.

◎ LIFE-ART PROCESS

In the Tamalpa Training of the San Francisco Dancers' Workshop, we have developed an approach we call a *life-art process*. Our intention is to use the body, movement, and the creative process as a metaphor for life, a way in which people can create a healthy, holistic way of life rather than a stereotyped system. People have an opportunity to apply this process to their unique individual and social needs. This process can be seen graphically in the chart (Figure 3–2).

At the very center of the large circles are two spirals. The spiral moving inward symbolizes deepened life experience—the personal life experience involved in the creative process. The spiral going out refers to the expanded art expression. The two interacting symbolize the life-art process of our dance movement approach. We are nourished by our life themes as they become the resources that we use to create our art. In the process of creating our art, we simultaneously transform and change; we grow in the life experience.

These three circles show the context through which we explore our resources. We begin by studying our bodies by experiencing and studying how the body moves. Then, by using the creative process, we create art experiences for ourselves. This is represented by the first circle outside the spirals. We organize our activities around developing awareness of what it is like to move, to have a body, and to create as an individual. We experience the differences when we take the same principles into relationship with one other person. We work in relationship to one or more people represented by the second circle in the chart. We have different life experiences when we are alone than we do when we are in a relationship. Movement relationships bring up many kinds of emotional factors as well as differing physical factors. We see the difference when we relate in a family-like configuration, dancing in relationship to two, three, or four people; dancing in a group; or dancing with a sense of a total community. We are always dancing in relationship to people in some way, and each type of relationship evokes its own expressive response.

We are always dancing in relationship to our physical environment, symbolized by the outermost circle. That environment may be an indoor or outdoor space; an urban space or a wilderness; a high place or a growth space; a nervous, anxious, smelly, noisy, congested,

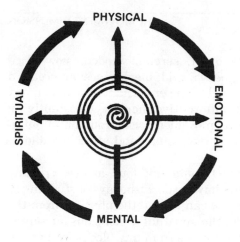

PHYSICAL

SPIRITUAL

EMOTIONAL

MENTAL

A UNIFIED APPROACH

DEEPENED LIFE EXPERIENCE

EXPANDED ART EXPRESSION

1. BODY/MOVEMENT & DANCE   2. PEOPLES   3. ENVIRONMENT

TECHNIQUES (partial list)

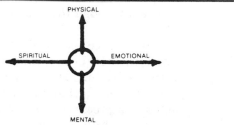

PHYSICAL
Anatomy & Kinesiology; Structural integration; Sequential Movements I, II, III; Movement exploration; Rhythmic & Movement Analysis; Space, Time & Force studies; Improvisation

EMOTIONAL
Gestalt Processes; 5 Part Process; Emotional Scripting; Attitudinal studies; Visualizations;

MENTAL
Theory; Journals; RSVP Cycles (Collective Creativity); Communication Skills; Scores

SPIRITUAL
Personal rituals; Social rituals; Environmental rituals; Meditation

PROGRESSIONS

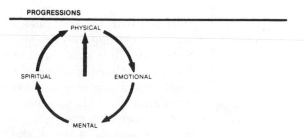

Figure 3–2.   A Life-Art Process.

automobile-dominated place; a quiet, serene, wooded, slow-paced place close to nature; a rugged, harsh, cold, bleak place; an ocean; a sandy beach; or a hot, tropical jungle. The environment has its many moods, and we respond to each differently. There is consistently an environmental context in dance movement. Environmental influences have tremendous impact on our beings and affect the dances we do.

Again referring to the chart, note the four arrows crossing through the circles. These arrows have to do with ways of studying so that we can isolate these areas: we can isolate the physical from the emotional from the mental from the spiritual dimensions ourselves. That isolation is done in order to free us from any blocks we have in any of those four areas. We reintegrate with the whole later in the process. We normally begin our work with the physical dimension and progress through the emotional, the mental, and then the spiritual areas.

We may be very weak in one area, so we isolate it in order to look into it further. In working through these progressions, we may use a variety of techniques, depending upon what people need and respond to most. These techniques, listed on the chart in each of the four major areas, are processes that we use to develop strength in these areas and to generate resources or material to work with. If a person is blocking just one area, emotional, for example, he or she is not going to be able to get through the progressions. So we choose the techniques that will help the person through this blockage. If a person has no ability or interest to order his or her inner material in a way that is communicable—in other words, is undeveloped in the mental area—and has become totally victimized by emotions or so carried away that the material has become totally subjective, then that person is not going to get through the progressions either.

Physical Area

We start with the body, and for that reason, we encourage people to learn everything they can about the body. They take anatomy and kinesiology. They study anthropologically the way they evolved this body, including the origin of the limbs, lungs, everything. We try to excite people about what an incredible wonder the body is. The body, after all, is the only way through which we can perceive the world. We also do sensory exercises. We take people out into a variety of settings—urban, seacoast, and wilderness environments—and stimulate the nervous system to alert the body and bring it more fully to life. So we emphasize learning both objective and subjective information about the body. We then begin with the very minute parts of movement, like the evolutionary processes of movement, starting with lying on the ground, as if going back to infancy, and gradually build to standing and moving through space. We work on the ground with our backs supported by the floor, and we learn simple releasing movements. We learn to *sense* the body. We learn the basic movements that the body can do through the spine and from the spine to other parts of the body—always in relationship to rhythm of the breath. We also work from the point of view of joint action and muscle contraction and release around the joint. We evolve from there to movement exploration, improvisation, ethnic life styles, and ways we can discover and develop our ability to have a sensitive moving body that is responsive to our expressive mind.

Emotional Area

Our method of taking people through the emotional area is a five-part process. We use the following system to help people identify where they are in terms of their emotional material and to learn to break through old patterns:[?]

1. *Identification*. The participants use movement, visualization, and dance scores to confront and identify old behavior patterns that are no longer effective.
2. *Release*. The participants break through the impasse by expressing the suppressed or frozen feelings associated with old patterns.
3. *Growth*. The participants use the material that is released in order to discover new potentialities and alternatives which they perform through dance.
4. *Transformation*. The participants apply what they have realized in their new dance to their everyday lives.
5. *Integration*. The participants have practiced a process that they can apply to the next impasse that they confront.

Suzanne's case is a good example of this five part process. Suzanne was able to identify something that could have been fatal. She came to us suffering from a throat tumor. She had been working in the program doing all the four areas and was using as her life theme her relationship with her parents. Her relationship with her father was especially critical. He had, in fact, died of a cancerous tumor in his throat. Suzanne carried a tremendous amount of tension in her own throat, as well as in her shoulders and part of her head and face.

Her movements were fluid enough in the rest of her body but were very stiff and unnatural in her neck area. Suzanne was holding back negative emotions.

Suzanne selected her father as her dance theme. That became part one—identification. She then did her dance but didn't confront the real problem at first. We could see that the dance was incongruent, that it was full of conflict. Suzanne's emotional stuckness was manifest in her throat because of her associations with her father; this led to a vulnerability to illness which had predisposed her to the throat tumor. What she had to do in going through the five-part process was go back to part one and confront the source of her inhibition, which was strong feelings about her father. She did work that allowed her to see all the ways she was carrying her relationship with her father into her life and into her other relationships, and she realized that she didn't need to do that.

This moved her into part two—the release phase of the process, and that's when healing began to take place. Suzanne went into intense rage, grief, and sadness. Days later, she went beyond the sadness and grew through a closure ritual done with others in the workshop. In this ritual, people were to find a place in the environment where they could be born and a place where they could die.

When Suzanne found her place, she experienced a sense of coming home—phase three. From there she began maturing and making choices in her life. She went into part four—transformation. At this level, she had a profound spiritual experience. Several months later, Suzanne's tumor had begun to disappear, and it ultimately disappeared altogether.

Mental Area

One of the techniques we use for working in the mental area is the RSVP cycle.[3] This cycle uses the basic elements of creativity. It allows for collective creativity yet provides a medium for each individual's output.

> R — *Resources* are what we have to work with. These include human and physical resources, such as experiences, events, and knowledge.
>
> S — *Scores* describe the activity leading to the performance. These are the details of the events that the performance is supposed to portray.

V — Valuaction analyzes the results of action and possible selectivity and decisions. The term *valuaction* was coined to suggest the orientation to values and action leading to positive non-judgmental attitudes. These may suggest improvements or additional activities to enhance the accuracy of the performance.

P — Performance is the *style* of implementing the score. After a *valuaction* is given to the resources, the score, and the quality of the performance, the score is recycled; that is, changes are made to create a more effective score—one that fulfills the original intentions. Then, the performance is done again.

Using the RSVP cycle, people develop the ability to be responsible and creative in producing tangible products. They learn from one another's differences, find new commonalities, and consequently expand their own vision. People learn to respect human differences, and they learn that people of all ages and all cultural or ethnic backgrounds have valuable input. They can enjoy full participation and share in decision making. They can take part in shaping their own art. The system is completely applicable to any activity we can possibly think of, not just in art but also in business, city planning, problem solving, or any human endeavor. Lawrence Halprin, who developed the RSVP cycle, says, "In a process-oriented society all the elements of creativity must be visible continuously, in order to work to avoid secrecy and the manipulation of people."

Spiritual Area

In any of the dances we work with—personal, social, environmental—powerful spiritual feelings are aroused within people. Qualities of consciousness come over us when we are aware of being part of something larger than ourselves, and we feel awed by the experience. Expression becomes like a totally mystic dance where there is some real connection experienced between us and a part of nature—human nature or the whole universe. One man did a dance that was a ritual of his love for a girl in the group, a love dance. Their relationship had just gone through a change, so he was expressing the love he still felt for her. He had put himself into such perfect harmony with all the elements around him—the physical environment, the woman, the people in the group—and his dance was coming from such a deep place within him, that he could have been any person at any time in history expressing a feeling that was universal. The experience is familiar to all of us, and it touches the same thing in each of us. It was as if the young man had done a dance which expressed something that we needed to have expressed, so we were made to feel a part of him at that moment.

Whether a simple movement or a complex myth, whenever the sense of connectedness with the whole is manifested, it evokes being part of a larger force than our individual selves. An awesome kind of "magic" is felt.

◎ DANCE AS HEALING

In applying a life/art process to dance, many relevant forms of dance can be created that respond directly and immediately to authentic situations of health and illness. An example of a form that a healing dance can take is a spontaneously drawn, life-sized portrait. Anna Halprin's portrait dance ultimately helped her to discover a contributing source of her illness.

> Three years after my operation (for a cancerous tumor, in the winter of 1972) I decided to create another life-sized self-portrait. I selected a place to work that was especially comforting to me. I went to the ocean, my favorite environment where I feel most relaxed and clear. I went alone and spent a week meditating, moving, and drawing my portrait. When it was all finished, I looked at it and it did not feel right. I saw my fantasy of myself and intuitively I knew I was hiding some realities. I turned it over and did my back side.

> All the time I was drawing on the back side of my portrait I was having internal bleeding. I experienced powerful physical and emotional reactions. I had fears of cancer returning. I knew, however, that I had a supportive community of friends and co-workers to be my witnesses.

> I returned home, called my doctor to report the symptoms of the bleeding, and was asked to go for tests. First, I called my group of friends, my family, and my co-workers and decided to dance my portrait immediately. Dancing my self-portrait was a marvelous experience for me. We have evolved a ritual for approaching this dance. No one is permitted to rehearse or plan ahead of time. Instead, each person is instructed to put their portrait up, stand before it, and wait until the dance within them begins to move; then follow the impulses and go with it wherever these feelings and movement responses will take them. I did just this. The first part, dancing my back side, was so full of violence, grief, and outrage that I was left weak and motionless, used up and finished. Then I did the front, more hopeful, side.

I felt my breath, and I imagined I was water and breath together. I imagined my breath was like a river that flowed through my body, out of it and into a huge sea. My arms and legs and head and chest and pelvis and backbone, my hands and feet, face, teeth, nose, tongue, my belly, my guts, all my insides seemed to flow with this water breath. It began moving with ease and smoothness, with fullness, increasing in range, turning me into spirals in space, transforming my voice into the sounds of chants. My friends and family joined with me in the chant as if their sounds were of the spontaneous song that nourished my spirit, that turned me, whirled me like a vortex in space. I felt at once both totally out of my body and yet deeply within. I experienced a glorious dance for myself, with the support of the others there with me. As a closure we all joined together in a circle. I felt relieved, calm, centered. I had my test after that, and there were no problems; the bleeding stopped. Yet I knew that I was not at all finished. The healing process needs to continue forever. I have more self-portraits to draw and perform; more visualizations to express on my journey to wholeness.[4]

When Anna took the material generated from this dance further, other aspects of herself were discovered, worked through, and expanded. She intuitively chose certain images that emerged from the self-portrait. The back side of the self-portrait was totally self-destructive; everything seemed impounded and black. She realized that she was emotionally stuck in a negative, self-deprecating place. Seeing her self-portrait was like looking at her own nightmare. Anna had invited her family, friends, and colleagues to witness the self-portrait dance so that she wouldn't avoid confronting the underlying problems. She finally had to face and feel the horror of her own ugliness, self-criticism, and self-disgust. The dance went on for three hours, bringing Anna from this negative place to a new level of realization and self-healing.

Anna had danced through her impasse, her inability to look at her ugly side. She believes that inability may have contributed in part to her susceptibility to cancer: she had repressed her ugly material and was not dealing with it. Anna was out of balance and, therefore, vulnerable to disease. She turned the portrait over and danced the other side and discovered the healing aspect of herself. After releasing the ugly part, she then needed to look at some of the positive aspects. She began by using the image of her breath as water, from an image of the ocean that she had drawn in her portrait. She used breathing as if it were the ocean and in this way was cleansing herself. That was four years ago.

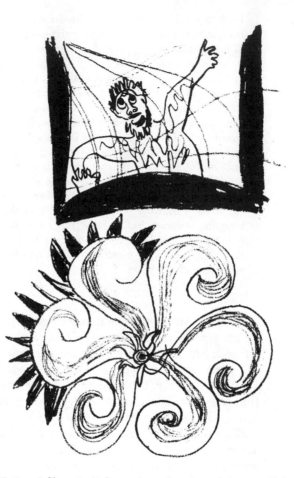

Figure 3–3.   Self-portrait drawn by a dance workshop participant.

Another example of a life-art dance is in Joseph's dance, performed recently. Joseph is a Native American. The life aspect of his dance was arrived at through a vision quest that he did for four days before performing his dance. A vision quest is a period of time spent in isolation in which a person seeks visions leading to insight. During the vision quest, Joseph fasted in a hut he made from pine branches. He was totally alone. The visions he found were of himself; he was confronting his own fears in the form of visions. No one knows what he or she will get when a vision quest is begun! Joseph was confronting his fear of the present and his anxiety of the future, among many other things. After he did his quest, he drew a portrait of himself. Then he danced that self-portrait. The self-portrait was the visualization of what he experienced in his vision quest; it was *who* he was in reality. The point is, Joseph's dance was not about some mythical character or an abstract concept; his dance was about himself. The self-portrait dance is a process that helps make the link between the inward and outward spirals. It helped Joseph sift out what was going on with himself and gave him the symbols to dance.

◎ INSIGHTS AND CONNECTIONS

By using the isolation of the physical, emotional, mental, and spiritual, we can arrive at a clear perspective of the areas that are weak or strong in our development. We can focus on areas that need to be strengthened and reintegrated later with a new and healthier attitude and wholeness in ourselves. An exciting aspect of the isolation-to-reintegration process is the many insights and connections we make.

The discovery of connections is made through a careful, sequential, step-by-step series of exercises that have been evolved in order to expose us to ourselves. There is a natural tendency to avoid using parts of ourselves that make us uncomfortable. By avoiding these uncomfortable areas, a lack of awareness results—it's as if those areas atrophy. So, by being led through a complete set of exercises designed to explore and uncover a total, ideal range of movement and/or emotions, we will notice parts of ourselves that we have cut off from awareness.

Betty noticed a connection when she wrote in her journal, "I was surprised at how tight my muscles felt when I tried to stretch in an open leg position. I also noticed that, when I did stretch in this position, some new feelings were aroused. I need to explore around this movement and find out what is going on."

With the guidance of a teacher, we may identify an area that has been unavailable, rigid, stuck, preventing healthy growth. We then begin the process of re-education and re-integration. We may find in the physical area, for example, that a movement range is extremely limited. Maybe someone is tight in their rib cage, or their shoulders are hiked up, or they have no awareness of their legs. These imbalances are evident as the person begins to expose himself or herself and explore within the range of physical material. The movement limitation will then come out in exercises that are aimed at getting in touch with emotional material, and the connections and limitations between the physical and emotional can be clearly seen and overcome.

A way to understand how we arrive at this information and how people who are in our program get at it is to understand that every session is carefully planned. There are specific exercises that people do together or individually or in smaller groups. Experiences, data, information, and exercises are presented according to the readiness of the group. Our exercises and process are aimed at discovering aspects of ourselves that can be creatively developed. Teachers need only be like co-witnesses with participants in the process of translating information from movement to understanding or insight.

Raised shoulders, for example, can indicate a range of emotional experiences or imprints that are problematical. We may be burdened by responsibilities and so have hiked our shoulders up in order to try to carry the burden; we may be shielding ourselves from a blow; or we may be holding back anger, holding back our shoulders from striking out at somebody. Sexual tension would be found in another area of the body—turned-in legs around the pelvis, for example, or a pelvis tilted back or forward.

The following case of a schizophrenic boy who came to our workshop points up the importance of the holistic approach. This was a smart young man. When he wanted to, he could communicate intelligently about many different things. This boy had an interesting aspect of spiritual development in his life. He had studied with a guru in India and had become deeply involved and even overwhelmed by the possibilities of his spiritual development. In some ways, he was overdeveloped in this area: after being in an ashram for a certain amount of time, he began developing a fantasy about being in touch with God. He held his eyes looking upward, and it became difficult for him to bring his eyes back down to a level where he could establish eye contact with people. No matter what he was doing, he maintained this meditative longing to be at one with God. He was not comfortable with being on the earth or in contact with human beings.

In the ashram, he had learned some meditation techniques for breath manipulation. These were somehow translated into holding his breath. We came to understand him through working with him, through observing his body and movements, and through noting the information he shared with us. He was blocked in physical expression and in emotional interactions with other human beings, so he was really almost split. His mental and spiritual areas were well developed, while his physical and emotional areas were almost totally undeveloped.

The young man was working in a dance movement workshop in which all of the other adults were normally functioning people. He sat off in the corner in his usual posture and wouldn't talk to anybody or look at anybody. In this workshop, we were using the technique of identifying ourselves through an animal fantasy, the animal we feel most akin to. When we identify on some fantasy level, we are sometimes able to release aspects of ourselves that we are embarrassed to express when we are closely tied to a social norm about ourselves. We began by drawing ourselves as the fantasy animal. He drew a picture of himself as a horse-like animal, with parts of his body sitting on top of a phallic-looking shape.

He danced the horse in himself, and eventually, he rode this horse in a repetitive movement that went on for 45 minutes. He rode around the room and over to other people. Gradually, his eyes dropped down, and he looked at people; he smiled and was receptive. By the end of the session, his shoulders had dropped, he was breathing normally, and his eyes had come down to a normal position. It made a big difference for him to move his shoulders and breathe normally. His second visualization drawing was amazing. He drew his entire body and a real horse instead of the disfigured sketch that included just a shadow of what we would recognize as a human body. When other people shared what happened for them in their animal fantasy, he was able to speak three or four fully coherent sentences and share his fantasy experience with the group.

In the workshop experience, he had something to do where all four levels of his being were appealed to in a way that was interesting to him. By being a horse, he was able to get into the physical aspect and experience the joy and satisfaction in physical activity. Movement, along with visualization and imagery, gave him a lively physical and emotional experience. During this experience, he was able to balance himself and relate to other people. Because he was so involved, he felt fully alive—functioning for himself as a social person. He needed this kind of balance and this sense of creativity, a sense of aliveness we all feel when we are creative in an active way.

◎ TAKING IT ALL HOME

As workshop participants go through the processes for physical, emotional, mental, and spiritual areas, they take responsibility to do the techniques in their terms after leaving the workshop. They may have an imprint, as the source of a problem, that is so strong it will take a lot of rehearsing to wash away; it is like a stain. Unless each person keeps this process going as a lifestyle, the problem usually comes back. Anna, for instance, had spent seven years trying to identify what brought about her illness. After her dance, she knew that she needed to maintain a balance in her lifestyle to remain creative and healthy. This balancing activity has to become a commitment in our lives, an agreement we make to ourselves that we understand this process and will use it.

After learning the process, people are encouraged to find their own personal ritual whereby they can live the kind of balancing process they've learned. We can live it in our relationships, in the kind of environments we create, everything. There is no sense in having it unless we apply it for ourselves. From the movement point of view, we can apply the process in our lives in the way we stand, the way we sit, and the attitude we carry in our bodies. Even while we are doing other activities, we can be aware of weaknesses or problems in certain areas and give them attention.

We can notice things when we drive the car. For example, we notice whether we are in a supported position or whether our shoulders are tensing up. We can scan our body from time to time to see if it is in the right alignment. Also, we can pay attention to the *quality* of exercise we get and know what works for our particular body and what we need to do for ourselves. We have the opportunity to learn something about our body and know what is the right diet of exercise for our body, just like we develop a sense of diet about food. We have seen the importance of stressing self-responsibility for this process in cases where the problems return if they're not given attention.

One example of a problem returning is a young woman who came to our workshop from Germany. She had not menstruated for 10 years. She had been to psychiatrists, doctors, and physiotherapists and had tried nearly everything. While she was participating in one of our trainings, we did a body reading that led her to identify an area of her body that made her confused and fearful—her pelvis. We used visualizations to "see" inside the pelvis. We asked her to imagine what it looked like. She could not imagine a thing; it was just black. So we painted the anatomical reality of what was in her pelvis. Then we moved the pelvis and explored the possible ranges. We guided her through flexion, extension, and rotation, while asking her to notice the articulation of the acetabula joint in this activity. We used anatomical references objectively until she was able to replace the black void in her pelvis with her own subjective visualizations. She danced the visualizations of these images and wrote in her journal all the feelings and stories that were aroused by this process.

The next day, we went to the oceanside and enacted the building of a village with a group of 25 people. While people were building the village, someone built a cave with bars on it using wooden sticks for bars. Hauled and dragged into the cave, the young German woman turned into an absolute monster. She was vicious as she acted out a demon that was possessing her. Soon, she broke through and came out of her cave; she was radiant! Everybody in the group did a sunset closure afterwards. One of the visualizations or images she used was imagining that her breath was the ocean; the ocean was playing a big part in this experience. The next day she menstruated.

We had guided this woman through all the integrative phases described earlier. She received a lot of support from her teachers and the group, but when she returned to Germany, she did not recreate the process for herself, nor did she have a support group. The problem returned.

She eventually came back for the training program where we could strengthen and deepen her understanding of the process. We worked with her on how she could take responsibility for creating the appropriate exercises that would maintain her harmony. She chose visualizations and movement as her main techniques and, through them, she found her emotional scripting. Ten years prior, when she was a teenager, she was terribly afraid of getting pregnant. Her body reacted to this fear by stopping menstruation. Understanding herself and using the techniques, she was able to confront and resolve the problem.

◎ INTEGRATING

Using physical movement alone as a therapy can be limiting if it is used in such a way that sensitivity and awareness of the whole movement process is cut off. In every muscle we have, there are sensory nerve endings, so there is no way that we can move our body without stimulating nerve impulses. Once stimulated, an impulse goes up into the brain through the thalamus, which then sends messages to different parts of the brain. These messages trigger off an acknowledgement of some kind; of a quality, a state of mind, an emotion, or an image. A person would have to be very out of harmony just to cut off that acknowledgement.

If we are lifting weights, "One, two, three, four," and our mind is totally goal oriented, and all we're thinking about is, "I'm going to do this movement for X number of times or do 10 leg kicks or I'm going to run for 6 miles," then there is no kinesthetic response to the movement. If we cut off the awareness of the sensation of the movement, it's just like repressing the whole nervous system. That awareness of the sensation is what connects all the other parts. Without this awareness in movement, it is possible to create an incredible amount of damage to the body.

A distinction can, therefore, be made between physical movement, as a purely goal-oriented kind of activity, and aware movement. Take that awareness and connection away and it is as if we are physically unconscious and are directing ourselves mentally, creating a split between movement and awareness—mind and body. Moving on a physical level with little or no awareness of our movement can lead to injury, whereas movement with emotional, physical, and mental awareness can lead to wellness and a rich enhancement in our lives.

Despite all of our work for balancing the individual and in bringing awareness to groups of people, we feel strongly that we can't be totally holistic or spiritual or healthy until our whole society has a sense of caring for one another and experiences a sense of connection and community. Imbalance still exists in our society—educationally, culturally, and economically.

We have much to learn from one another's differences; from the Asian, the Black, the Native American, and the Chicano communities. All diversity is important. We developed a special Reach Out program that has been in existence for 10 years. We are situated in a mixed community in San Francisco, and we draw local residents from a variety of ethnic backgrounds. These people participate in a workshop that enables them to tap the rich resources of their heritage and reaffirm themselves from this focus. Participants have the opportunity to see their own special ways of expressing themselves, of being in the world, and taking pride in their own cultural heritage. The workshop provides a place for them to express and explore that heritage. For example, in one movement piece, an Oriental woman used an ancient Chinese wedding custom, involving preparations for a marriage ceremony, as a base for "scoring" a dance of a young woman's rite of passage into adulthood. The colorful result was not merely an enactment of an ancient ritual but also a remembering of undeniable cultural influences that have significance for today's female human events.

We feel that the answer to equality is not the "melting pot" idea of conformity. We feel it is important to maximize and respect our differences and arrive at new commonalities. In this way, we can become more appreciative and supportive of one another and evolve a dynamic, authentic, healthy community.

◎ CONCLUSION

Through development of the capacity to move with awareness can emerge a new and positive approach to health, improved interpersonal relations, and community and environmental development. This can take place with a diversity of participants—people of all ages, ethnic, and cross-cultural backgrounds. Mohair, an Israeli Arab who studied this approach in the Tamalpa Training, has returned to Jerusalem, where he is directing a theatre group of Arabs and Jews that gives performances and workshops for Arab and Jewish children as a way to promote trust and understanding between the two groups. Carolyn, a former city planner, uses her experiences with the movement processes to teach movement to elders in her community. A traditional nurse, who became intensely involved with the visualization material, has left her old job to retrain and specialize in the use of movement and visualization for cancer patients. A young man, who is an athletic director in a high school, is incorporating this "no win, no lose" approach into his athletic department. In a religious setting, the movement process was used to collaborate with members of a synagogue. The rabbi and cantor, along with dancers, re-examined the Friday night *shabot*. Stereotypes and old imprints were replaced with new and meaningful ways to express joy, release, and celebration. People of the city of San Francisco participated in a collective dance to honor the sunrise that began on Twin Peaks; journeyed throughout the day in neighborhoods, subways, and public squares; and ended at the ocean with a sunset ceremony. The dancers evoked a unique spirit, the best visions, and a healthy environment for their community.

The list is exciting and endless. We can see a new holistic attitude beginning to permeate our lives, and we can see dance as a universal form, a powerful force in shaping human experience. We all know that, throughout history, people have continually danced their most profound needs and struggles as a means to reaffirm harmony with the natural and spiritual forces. Now, once again, we have the wonderful possibility of applying the creative process to make dances with deep transforming power. Dances based on people's common experiences, when expressed and enjoyed, are signs of a creative, healthy, and unified community. The forming and performing of these dances is a means of creating and nourishing a community of people.

REFERENCES

1. Margaret H'Doubler, *Dance, A Creative Art Experience* (New York; F.S. Crofts and Company, Inc., 1940).

2. Anna S. Halprin with James Hurd Nixon, "Dance as a Self-Healing Art" (San Francisco Dancers' Workshop, 1977).

3. Lawrence Halprin, *The R.S.V.P. Cycles* (New York: George Braziller, Inc., 1969).

4. Halprin and Nixon, *op.cit.*

4

THE MERIDIAN
DIMENSION

PROFESSOR
JACK R. WORSLEY,
M.Ac., Dr.Ac. (China), F.C.C.Ac., F.O.M.C.

The meridian system of the human body is the working area of traditional Chinese acupuncture, the system of medicine that originated in China between four and five thousand years ago. The meridians are energy pathways that encompass the body, and the Chinese hold that it is the condition of the energy flowing through the meridians that determines our state of being. This chapter is an account of the traditional Chinese way of viewing and treating the physical, mental, and spiritual features that constitute an individual. Without some knowledge of this perspective, the role of the meridians cannot be understood.

As a method of treatment, it must, of course, be remembered that acupuncture is one system among many, each of which has the same object of maintaining health. Accordingly, when we describe the way in which the acupuncturist views and treats his patient, we shall be describing a particular form of interaction that can subsequently be compared directly and illuminatingly with other systems of therapy described in this book. But, at first, the following commentary must necessarily be regarded as describing a unique and exclusive system. We shall be discussing the concepts by which acupuncturists, and Taoists generally, describe and account for the human being as a dynamic unity within the greater unity of the universe. In this description, the role of *ch'i* energy, its highways through the body (the meridians), and its qualitative changes in response to the movements of the environment is quite fundamental. It would not be meaningful to place these concepts along side other, more familiar concepts that describe the constitutive systems of the body as we know it and to build up in that way a picture of a network of cooperating parallel processes. *Ch'i* energy should not be regarded as a constituent of the body in the same way that blood is, however much it may appear, to a superficial glance, that acupuncturists try to manipulate it by hydrodynamic engineering. The system of meridians is not an extra anatomical fact comparable, for instance, to the nervous system. The position, rather, is that *ch'i* energy and its pathways are an alternative way of viewing the human being, both within himself and within the totality in which he exists. What is being asked of the reader is that he should assimilate the following account as if it were the description of an unknown territory, not as something he should repeatedly evaluate by relating it to similar-sounding bits of descriptions he is already familiar with.

◎ *CH'I* ENERGY

Ch'i energy suffuses the entire universe. It is the essence of a thing, the essential energy that gives it being and form, and it is because of this all-pervading energy that there is an interaction between human beings and the physical world. An energy change in one will reflect in the energy of the other but not necessarily by a mechanical causal effect. The traditional Chinese say that, in order to understand health and disease in the individual, we must learn to understand the subtle effects of nature—the effects of the different climates, the seasons, the daily cycle, and the effects of thoughts, mood, and lifestyle.

◎ *YIN* AND *YANG*

Yin and *yang* are concepts that describe the two poles of the dualities that exist in nature. In Chinese cosmogony, it is the fact of these polarities in natural phenomena that allows for attraction, repulsion, movement, and change. Originally, *yin* meant the shady side of a mountain and *yang* the sunny side, but their use was extended so that *yin* came to stand for everything dark, contractive, cold, receptive, and supportive, and *yang* came to stand for everything light, expansive, hot, active, and transforming. These dual principles not only characterize every aspect of existence, they also describe cyclic change, such as night and day, contraction and expansion, or decay and growth, where *yin* and *yang* continually change from one to the other. The *ch'i* energy, as it flows from one meridian to the next, undergoes a continual transformation in quality from *yin* to *yang* within the body itself and within the context of environmental shifts. The acupuncturist, noting these rhythmic changes, can use this understanding in planning a treatment.

◎ THE LAW OF THE FIVE ELEMENTS

The next continuous cycle in creation that the Chinese have observed is a series of five successive modes which continually give way to one another. Their names have not been left in transliterated Chinese— as with *yin* and *yang* or *ch'i*—but translated into English. Such attempts at translation run into difficulties at the present time, since these concepts are still unfamiliar to the modern Western mind. As we use them and begin to understand and appreciate them, however, the words we now employ to carry this range of ideas become enlarged in meaning in order to accommodate the ideas. So, bearing in mind this extension of meaning, we will now consider the five elements. Each is called after an actual material substance or principle, but it would be misleading to tie down the qualities encompassed by one element to the specific qualities of the physical substance, or principle that lends the element its name. The elements are metal, water, wood, fire, and earth, and they refer, in the case of a human being, as much to mental and spiritual qualities as to the physical body. The system is intended to reflect the fact that the *ch'i* energy, as it undergoes its myriad transformations, takes on five elemental qualities that jointly define the qualitatively diverse nature of phenomena.

There are two principal interrelated cycles: the first is the creative, or *shen* cycle, where the energy of one element gives way to the next; and the second is the control, or *k'o* cycle, in which the energy of one element checks that of another. The five elements in the cycle are shown in Figure 4–1.

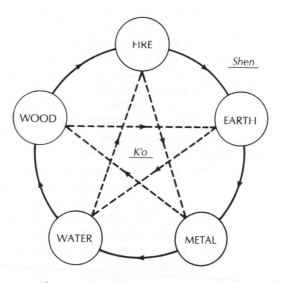

Figure 4–1. The *Shen* and *K'o* cycles.

The five elements are expressed in the different aspects and constituents of a person: in each organ, each sense organ, each body tissue, each body fluid, each emotion, each sound of the voice, each mental state, and so on. Their interrelations are complex, and there are several cycles of transformation that operate in different contexts.

◎ THE MERIDIAN SYSTEM

Ch'i energy is everywhere in the body, but the meridians are like reservoirs of *ch'i*, each with a specific sphere of influence. There are 12 principal meridians, each with a superficial pathway lying close to the surface of the body and a network of deep pathways that connect it to underlying structures, internal organs, and other meridians. The acupuncture points lie along the superficial pathways of each of the meridians, and they provide the most accessible arena in which acupuncturists can reach and effect the *ch'i* energy. The acupuncture points will be described in greater detail when we have looked at more of the factors that determine their use.

In a shorthand used by acupuncturists, each of the 12 meridians is known by the name of a major associated internal organ or physical function. Each meridian comes within the domain of one of the five elements. Thus, in earth we have the spleen and stomach meridians; in metal, the lung and colon; in water, the kidneys and bladder; in wood, the liver and gall bladder; and in fire, the heart, small intestine, circulation-sex, and three-heater meridians. These names are appropriate as far as they go, but, as we pointed out in the case of the names of the elements, they fall far short of communicating the full significance of the characteristics of each meridian. In a much deeper and broader sense, which the traditional acupuncturist has to bear in mind as he uses these limited terms, each meridian is associated with a specific range of administrative operations or functions. The description of the mechanism of these operations forms a physiological picture quite unknown in the West. To explain their workings, the Chinese have made an analogy between the functions of the 12 meridians and the functions of 12 ministers or officials. Each "official" is in charge of a sphere of activity that he or she alone can perform and which is essential to the work and well-being of all the other officials. If one of them falls sick, this puts a strain on all the others. When they are all performing their tasks correctly, however, the triple realm of body, mind, and spirit is integrated and comes to full maturity.

In restoring and promoting the healthy balance of *ch'i* energy in the meridians, the acupuncturist has to contact and question each of the officials in the patient.

The names of the officials of the meridians are as follows (the descriptions are taken from *The Yellow Emperor's Classic of Internal Medicine*):

Meridian	*Number*	*Official*
Heart	I	The supreme Controller: the official who excels through insight and understanding.
Small Intestine	II	The Controller of the transformation of matter: the official who separates the pure from the impure.
Bladder	III	The Controller of the storage of fluid: the magistrate of a region that stores fluid.
Kidney	IV	The Controller of fluid: the official who does energetic work and excels by his ability and cleverness.
Circulation-sex	V	The external Protector of the heart: the official who is the source of joy and pleasure.
Three-heater	VI	The Official of the three burning spaces: the commander of all energies—the energy of the upper, middle, and lower divisions; the inside and outside; and the left and right sides of the body.
Gall Bladder	VII	The Official of decisions and judgement: the true and upright official who excels in making decisions and judgement.
Liver	VIII	The Official of planning: the military leader who excels in his strategic planning.
Lung	IX	The Controller of receiving *ch'i*: the official of rhythmic order.
Colon	X	The Controller of the drainage of dregs: The official who propagates the right way of living and who generates evolution and change.
Stomach	XI	The Controller of rotting and ripening: the official of the public granaries who grants the five tastes.
Spleen	XII	The Official of the transport of energy: the official who distributes nourishment.

◎ SIGNALS OF DISEASE

Health in the individual is reflected in a balanced flow of *ch'i*, in good quality, throughout the meridians. For most of us, leading what is generally held to be a normal way of life, this represents an unlikely ideal. Our *ch'i* energy is susceptible to stresses and strains, trauma, and pollution. Generally, we can deal with temporary imbalances arising from difficult periods of our lives, or we find a way to compensate for imbalances that we cannot overcome. It is when an imbalance is causing us serious distress, or interfering in the realization of our potential, that we need to seek some form of help.

The acupuncturist will strive to see his patient, not as he is at the time of examination, but as he would be if he were well and whole. The personality and behavior of a person when ill will not necessarily be true to his real nature, but this very disequilibrium will provide important clues as to the specific features of the imbalance. The surest and most informative clues to imbalance come from a highly developed method of pulse diagnosis, but, in fact, every aspect of a person's presence is a manifestation of the quality of his energy.

Most internal conditions do not develop overnight. The body has a remarkable facility for giving out warning signals long before a state of imbalance has developed to the stage of clinical symptoms. We are all familiar with the mild aches and pains, which warn us that we need to slow down or smoke fewer cigarettes, or with a feeling of mental unease, which makes us aware that we need to re-examine our life situation. Similarly, whenever the energy flow in one of the meridians becomes unbalanced, we begin to manifest certain signs that are specific to that meridian. Among these signs are particular colors, sounds, emotions, and odors, and each one has an association with one of the five elements.

An interesting fact about Chinese medicine and philosophy is that there is no value difference between having too much or too little of a thing. Both are equally off track and equally disturbing. The Chinese aim for harmony, equilibrium, and balance. The acupuncturist must learn to divest the words "plus" and "minus" of their usual connotations.

When we look at a person's face, we see certain hues showing particularly around the temples and the mouth. In health, we show a balance of the five colors: white, blue, green, red, and yellow. But if, say, a person has an imbalance of the kidney meridian, connected with the element water, then we see either an excess of blue or a total absence of blue in these areas. This is irrespective of skin tone. Looking around a room full of people, we see many who have a similar skin tone but show very different colors in these areas of their faces. Some of the colors are easier for some people to see than others, and some can cause a bit of a problem even to an experienced acupuncturist. A total lack of red is often rather similar to white, although the lack of red tends to be more grey and highlight the presence of other colors, while white will shine out more clearly. These colors are important diagnostic clues, and they also give feedback as to improvement following a treatment, when they will change within seconds. They are not easy to see, and this skill requires many years of development of visual sensitivity.

As a meridian becomes imbalanced, we also notice a change in the expression of a person's voice. The five relevant sounds of a voice are weeping, groaning, shouting, laughing, and singing. We may find either a predominance of one sound, expressed out of context, or a marked lack of the sound when it would be appropriate. For instance, the person who is always laughing when there is really nothing at all funny to laugh about is saying, "Please help my heart, circulation-sex, small intestine, or three-heater meridian." Conversely, the same is true of the person who never laughs when his life is full of things to laugh about.

Besides color and sound, emotions are important keys, Here we consider grief, fear, anger, joy, and sympathy. All have their appropriate place in day-to-day life. We are emotive beings, and we are influenced by many factors that will arouse anger, fear, laughter, and so on. But occasionally, we meet someone whose anger is really predominant. In fact, for the purposes of diagnosis, it is not enough to stop at that. We must try to establish the type of anger. We know that anger is associated with wood, but each of the elements is composed of all five elements, and an inappropriate anger may be the result of an imbalance of wood within any of the elements. Is it a stubborn, cold type of anger—the kind where you wish that the person would come out and do something or the kind where you get the feeling that, at any moment, he might put a knife in your back? Or is it the type of anger in which a person goes around upsetting as many people as possible and is always confronting: "What did you say that for?" or "Why are you doing it like that?" He has to get his anger out; he picks fights or kicks the cat. In the first instance, it is an anger from metal, an imbalance of wood within metal. The second case is a straightforward wood within wood type of anger.

Earth anger manifests in the person who feels deprived. These people need sympathy and yet they reject it and are angry when it is offered. Generally, they get angry with themselves, and when they get really angry, they often dissolve in tears. They are very unstable, and out of contact with the earth, and they will tend to disintegrate, just as a child, when deprived of its mother, will eventually burst into tears.

It is only when an emotion is expressed out of context that it has any diagnostic value. For example, we expect to see grief in the event of a loss, but, as with the other emotions, grief has a natural time span, and we would not expect to see someone overcome by this emotion years after the event.

The five odors are a little easier to work with in that an odor will either be present in connection with an imbalance or absent in health. The odors are not from perspiration. They will disappear or change dramatically, in an instant, after treatment. The five odors are rotten, putrid, rancid, scorched, and fragrant. Possibly the scorched smell that accompanies a fever is the most familiar to us. At one time, it was quite common for a Western physician to use odor as part of his diagnostic armory.

We must realize that these diagnostic signals are subtle and take many years to master. They are, nonetheless, objective and reveal much information about the state of balance of the meridians. The traditional Chinese abhorred surgical cuts into the body, and their system of medical diagnosis is built on a keen observation of external appearances.

> By observing the external symptoms one gathers knowledge about internal disturbances. One should watch beyond the ordinary limits for what is unfit and inadequate. One should observe the minute and trifling things as if they were of normal size, and when they are then treated they cannot become dangerous.

> To treat and to cure disease means to examine the body, the breath, the complexion, its glossiness or degree of moisture, and the pulse, as to whether it is flourishing or deteriorating and whether the disease is a recent one. But then the actual treatment must follow, for later on there is no time.[1]

These quotations are taken from the *Huang-ti Nei-ching Su-wen*, which is the extant text of *The Yellow Emperor's Classic of Internal Medicine*. This is the most important classical textbook of Chinese medicine. It was first written down in about 400 BC. The book was written in the form of a dialogue between the Yellow Emperor, Huang Ti, and his court physician Ch'i Po. It is a treatise on physiology, pathology, diagnosis and prognosis, diet, and therapy, as well as philosophy, politics, and ethics. It sets out the theory on which acupuncture is based.

◎ OTHER DIAGNOSTIC FACTORS, THE ENERGETIC CYCLES

In health, there is a balance of *yin* and *yang* in our day-to-day life. A period of greatly accelerated activity needs to be followed by a period of withdrawal and calm: a chill needs to be followed by a fever, for a person to reach a state of balance. But, if imbalance arises in this cycle, an excess of *yin* will result in cold, numb, paralyzing, aching diseases, while an excess of *yang* will result in hot, sensitive, acute, and painful diseases. An imbalance within this dyad can be corrected through the meridian system. Unfortunately, the process is not simple, since *yin* exists within *yang* and *yang* within *yin*. The cause of an excess of *yang* may be overabundant *yang* within *yang* or deficient *yin* within *yang*. The traditional diagnosis is all-important in establishing the correct approach to treatment.

The next most important energetic cycle is, of course, the five elements. Each season is an expression of an element: spring is wood, summer is fire, late summer (harvest time) is earth, autumn is metal, and winter is water. When our energy is in balance, we find joy and beauty in all the seasons and climates, and a particular yearning for one, or loathing for another, is informative in acupuncture diagnosis. A seasonal variation in symptoms is also indicative of a specific area of imbalance. An obvious case is hay fever, which is commonly aggravated in the spring or late summer and more rarely in high summer, autumn, and winter. Some people find that feelings of anxiety become exaggerated during the spring or autumn, depending on the meridian that is the primary cause.

When treating a patient, we must observe the seasons and attend to the proper things in each season. Grass does not grow in winter, and to some extent, neither do we. When treating a person with chronic tissue damage, it may well be that we have to wait until spring to see a great deal of activity and new growth in his body.

The different climates have a resonance with our five elements. A person with an imbalance in one of the fire meridians may feel much better or much worse in the warmth of the sun. Similarly, the radiations of different colors affect our energy. The five principal colors connected with the elements are white, blue, green, red, and yellow. We find people who love green or hate yellow. They say the color doesn't suit them. In fact, when a patient begins to wear a color he has avoided for years, we almost don't need to ask him how he is. Aubergine is the one color that supports all the elements, irrespective of the type of imbalance.

It is an interesting fact that, when an imbalance is in its early stages, a person will crave the color, season, climate, taste, and emotional situations that will support his energy and encourage health. In more serious cases of imbalance, we find that a person will seek out those things that encourage imbalance and, in the end, promote greater distress. For example, in the early stage of an imbalance of the kidney meridian, extra salt in the diet will help the kidneys, but, as the imbalance proceeds, salt becomes harmful to the condition and yet is more strongly craved.

Our energy varies with the daily twenty-four-hour cycle. Each meridian has a two-hour period when its energy is at a peak and its associated functions are most active. Twelve hours later, it has a period of lowest energy and most rest. These two-hourly changes are tied to the motion of the sun rather than to our working hours. This fact is significant and tends to become overlooked. The peak time for the eliminative system of the body is between 5 and 7 a.m. To get someone up at this time in the morning can often be enough to help a case of chronic constipation. Of course, we accumulate as many toxic and polluted thoughts in our minds as toxins in our bodies, and it may help someone to feel clearer and lighter mentally if he exercises his eliminative processes during this peak time.

The peak time for the stomach meridian is from 7 to 9 a.m., which makes us appreciate the importance of having a good breakfast and which makes our tendency to have a large meal at the end of a working day seem rather foolish. One difficulty is that 7 to 9 p.m. is the peak time for the circulation-sex meridian, which is the meridian most concerned with interpersonal relationships, warmth, and joy, and we have a habit of combining conviviality with overeating.

Sometimes a person's habits give direct insight into the state of his or her meridians. Many people who suffer with insomnia find that they cannot go to sleep until after 3 a.m. In most cases, this is due to a hyperfunctioning liver meridian, particularly if there is a heavy drug history. But, as usual, it is important to remember that each person is different, and it may be that this pattern is due to a malfunction of the small intestine meridian, which has its low time from 1 to 3 a.m. There are people who wake at 3 a.m. and cannot go back to sleep until light comes with the dawn. This fact signals the lung meridian. Or they may wake between 3 and 5 a.m. with an urgent need to pass water, which then clues us into the bladder meridian, since this is the time of its lowest energy when it is normally resting. When these patterns change with treatment, we know that the energy of the meridians is coming into balance.

As we have seen, each meridian is associated with one particular range of functions in a person, and it would be instructive here to consider briefly the official in charge of one of the meridians, since it is through the officials that we can make sense of the different aspects of the person that are linked by association with one meridian and one element.

The liver meridian has a special connection with the eyes and vision, ligaments and coordinated movement, and anger and self-assertion. The official of the liver meridian is called the Planner, and it is associated with the wood element—the element of birth, growth, and development. A person with a healthy Planner will have good vision, both literally, in the sense of eyesight, and figuratively, in the sense of vision of the future. A severely imbalanced liver meridian tends to be reflected in feelings of resignation, despair, and hopelessness, since the person cannot see the possibility of a future or of further growth and development. This may be accompanied by any of a whole range of physical symptoms. Some disturbance of the vision is quite common, e.g., foggy vision, floating spots, gritty eye, or bad focus.

A person may be driven to compensate for insufficient plans by becoming inflexible and rigid, and it is not unusual for this to manifest in the person's physical body as a lack of coordination, a rigidity in the ligaments, inertia, and paralysis.

At this point, the reader may well be beginning to think that almost any physical symptom can probably be explained in terms of bad planning, and, to some extent, this is true. The key to the problem is to consider the whole person. If a tightening and stiffening of the ligaments is associated with a mental inability to plan, then we may be confident that the cause of the problem is the liver official. If, on the other hand, we find someone who is afraid to move, who feels swamped and overwhelmed by other people, whose mental processes are disjointed and abrupt, then we would expect that the rigidity in the ligaments came from a lack of fluid in the tissues, and we would investigate the kidney official, the official who controls fluids and fluidity and is associated with the element water and with fear.

It is important to assess the state of the planning official in every patient, even when it is not the primary area of imbalance, to ensure that the person is able to plan for the transition from sickness to health and then to maintain his health.

◎ STRESS

A major difference between acupuncture and Western medicine is that acupuncture is not so much concerned with the present condition of an organ as with the state of energy associated with it. Once the energy has become seriously imbalanced, we know that, in time, the person will start to manifest distress signals in the form of mental and physical symptoms. The task of the acupuncturist is to establish the initial area of imbalance in response to stress which has led, by however long and complicated a route, to the collection of symptoms that now brings the patient to his surgery.

The Chinese are quite specific in their analysis of the types of stress that may initially bring about imbalance. There are two categories. The first concerns the external causative factors of disease, which consist of climatic conditions, such as excessive exposure to heat, cold, damp, dryness, and wind and of mechanical and chemical injuries. The second comprises the internal factors, which are mainly emotional. These include excessive fear, anger, grief, or continuous lack of joy and any congenital factors. It is only when our resistances have been lowered by one of these agents that we become susceptible to infection by bacteria, viruses, parasites, and so on. This is one of the reasons why not everyone will succumb in an epidemic.

At this time in modern society, most people are quite well insulated from the extremes of our environment, excepting accidents, and a large percentage of disease is a result of the internal causative factors. Sometimes the causative agent will stand out quite clearly, but more often, we find a history of a succession of stresses. In either case, the acupuncturist must isolate the meridian that is in the most need of help, although it is likely that several meridians will need support and tending in order to direct the person towards health.

TRADITIONAL DIAGNOSIS

The aim of the traditional diagnosis is to ascertain the state of the person's twelve officials, five elements, and *yin/yang*. It is this information that tells us where help is needed, not the symptoms. Each patient has arrived at his present situation by a unique path. Although we may find a dozen people with the same label to their symptoms, they will reveal a dozen different diagnoses and require a dozen different treatment plans. When we enhance, balance and harmonize the *ch'i* energy at the appropriate level—physical, mental, or spiritual—we know that the sufferer will begin to function better. If the condition has not gone so far that all the natural healing powers of the person cannot reverse it, then healing will occur, and the symptoms will disappear.

The acupuncturist uses four approaches to diagnosis: seeing, asking, listening, and feeling. He observes the condition of the body, the posture, the gait and mannerisms, and, of course, the colors on the face. He asks about the background of the trouble, about symptoms, and about personal and family history. Meanwhile, he must listen to the sound of the patient's voice as well as to what is said. He does a physical examination and assesses the texture of the skin; variations in temperature; the condition of the hair, nails, and eyes; and notes the odor and reads the pulses.

The Pulses

An acupuncturist reads the pulses in six different positions along the radial artery of each wrist. These 12 pulses are not the same as the radial pulse monitored by a Western physician. Each pulse corresponds to one of the 12 meridians and gives information as to the quantity and quality of the energy flow within it. The ability to read the pulses requires many years of training and experience, but a skilled acupuncturist can read the medical history and prognosis of a patient from the pulses alone. Pulse reading is done throughout an acupuncture treatment to monitor the patient's response, since the pulses change within seconds of needling.

> The feeling of the pulse is the most important medium of diagnosis. . . . Nothing surpasses the examination of the pulse, for with it errors cannot be committed.[2]

Pulse reading is complicated by the fact that the energy level in a meridian varies according to the season and the time of day, and these must be taken into consideration before we decide whether a pulse is indicating an imbalance or not. Imbalances become apparent in the pulses long before an actual illness is manifested in the body.

The aim of the diagnosis is to find the acupuncture point that will unlock the imbalance of energy and set in process a series of changes which will eventually restore balance to each of the meridians. This is the ideal treatment, known as the *Su-wen* or "one-needle treatment." With most people, however, their energy picture is such that they require more protracted attention to set them on a course to health.

◎ TREATMENT

There are about 1000 acupuncture points in all, with about 360 in common use. Every point will affect the whole person, but treatment may be directed more to one level than another, depending on the point and the needle technique. A point may be selected to encourage a rebalancing of the five elements or to clear a blockage in a pathway, to bring assistance to an official, or to revitalize the spirit. Often, the name of a point gives an indication of when it might be used: spirit path, spirit burial ground, heavenly fountain, palace of weariness, thought dwelling, bubbling spring, *yang* support, happy calm, bright and clear. There are points which are gates—gate of hope, dark gate, cloud gate, lubrication food gate—and points that are gutters and ditches and good for cleansing—meridian gutter, insect ditch.

The reader may wonder how it is that intervention by something as gross as a needle will allow change to occur in such fine aspects of a person as the mind and spirit. The answer is that we are dealing with energy, and the needle is merely an instrument to contact a person's energy. The needles are very fine, nearly as fine as the hair on one's head. Depending on the nature of the energy imbalance, the needle, which is inserted to the depth of the energy flow, may be manipulated and withdrawn within a second or two or manipulated and left in for five to twenty minutes or even longer if necessary. The person may experience some sort of sensation as the needle is manipulated, which can be anything from a feeling of heat or numbness to a slight ache or pulling in the area of the point or at some other place further along the meridian pathway.

Besides the use of needles, the acupuncturist has a technique called *moxibustion* to warm and revitalize sluggish and cold energy. A little cone of a dried, pulverized herb, *moxa*, is placed on the surface of the body at the acupuncture point and is lit so that it smolders. It is removed when the patient begins to feel its warmth and long before the possibility of scarring. Sometimes it may be burnt on the handle of a needle, which then allows the warmth to be carried deep into the body.

How quickly a person responds to treatment is a very individual matter. A lot depends on the severity of the disease, the length of time that the patient has suffered from it, the drugs that have been and are being taken, and so on. Occasionally, a chronic condition will respond very rapidly to treatment, but this is rare. When an illness is deep seated in the body, it generally takes time for the natural processes to be revived, do their work, and rectify the trouble. A patient is not expected to cut down on prescribed drugs until his physician decides that there is sufficient improvement in his mental or physical condition.

In general, patients will be treated once a week until they are holding their improvement, and then they will need treatment once every 14 days, once a month, once every turn of the season, and finally, once a year as a precaution to monitor that they are maintaining good health.

Responses to acupuncture treatment follow the same healing laws as other systems of natural medicine. To effect a cure, disease must travel from within to without, from above to below, and symptoms must return in the reverse order from that in which they came.

As an example, let us consider the hypothetical case of a patient who, as a child, develops eczema, which is suppressed at the age of 10. Because of the intimate connection between the skin and lungs, this suppression leads to asthma at the age of 14. At 20, she develops menstrual disorders and, at 34, comes to have treatment for neuralgia. During the course of treatment, as the neuralgia clears, we will expect a temporary flare-up of the menstrual problems, followed by a short spell of asthma, or some sort of chest condition, and finally a recurrence of some sort of skin rash. We would do nothing to treat the menstrual disorder, asthma, or skin rash, since we know that they will only last a short time and are a necessary step in effecting a cure. In fact, this example is more true to a blackboard discussion than a real situation since life is always more complicated. The past symptoms can come back in many guises, even to the extent that a period of mental depression may come back on the physical level or vice versa.

A person may experience a temporary aggravation of symptoms immediately after a treatment, followed by an improvement. This is an encouraging sign that the condition is responding to treatment and may be helped or cured. As aspects of a person that have been malfunctioning for months or years are reawakened or, if necessary, calmed down, the person is bound to experience a temporary period of discomfort followed by an increased feeling of well being.

Case Histories

Two patients arrived, both presenting complaints of migraine headaches. The first, a woman of 42, arrived 20 minutes early for her appointment. She was carefully dressed, had a greenish look to her complexion, and addressed the receptionist in a loud, barking voice, asking if her practitioner would be ready to receive her on time, what she could read about acupuncture while she was waiting, and whether she could make an exact schedule of future appointments.

In relating her history, she explained that she suffered from one-sided headaches that occurred regularly every eight or nine days. Chocolate, alcohol, or fatty foods, however, would bring them on immediately, and she was particularly susceptible to stormy weather.

The headaches began with a feeling of nausea and a disturbance in her vision, and, as the pain intensified, she needed to lie down in a dark room free of noise. Medication, taken soon enough, somewhat reduced the level of pain. She also complained that the whole of her right side felt "dead" relative to her left side, but that neurological tests had revealed no reason for this.

Her headaches began in her teens, six months after she moved to a new school—having been faced with a choice, which seemed to have troubled her, of moving to a new town with her parents or remaining in her old school and staying with friends. Following school, she had various jobs and then married and started a family. Her husband walked out on her five years ago, leaving her with two children (now aged nine and twelve). The dead feeling in her body began at this time, and so did a problem of insomnia. (She was rarely able to go to sleep before 1 or 2 a.m., and she felt permanently tired.) It was at this time, too, that the incidence of migraine attacks increased.

The traditional acupuncture examination and pulse diagnosis showed that she had a severe imbalance in the wood element, involving both the gall bladder meridian, which is connected with coordination and the ability to make decisions, and the liver meridian, which is connected with the ability to make plans. She volunteered, in fact, that several times in her life, she felt she had made "the wrong decision" but that she had not had enough self-confidence to act otherwise. Whenever she thought of her husband now, she had bouts of furious anger, though she could accept in her "more rational moments" that she had been very difficult to live with. She said that her husband had caused her constant irritation by unpunctuality and his refusal to state exactly what his daily arrangements would be. She had felt unable to control her need to overplan his life, and now the same pattern was arising with the children. Furthermore, she now felt that she was living in the past, and it frightened her to consider her life in the future.

After her first few acupuncture treatments, the feeling of "deadness" in her right side disappeared. She said also that she had had an experience which she could only describe as a "divine revelation," when, for the first time, she felt free from feelings of guilt about her husband and clearer about how to handle arrangements between himself and herself about the children.

Over the next period of treatments, she described an increasing feeling of self-confidence, easier relations with her children, an improvement in her sleeping pattern, and an increase in her energy level and ability to face the world. As the wood element—the element of birth, rebirth, and growth—came into balance, her natural abilities gradually reasserted themselves. She began to make arrangements to take a part-time job while her children were at school. Meanwhile, her migraine headaches continued in the same pattern. After 12 weekly treatments, her migraines started to appear about every 16 days. Her treatments were then spaced to every two weeks, then to once a month, and the following spring, after nine months of treatment, her migraines stopped altogether.

The second patient was a young man of 30. He was wearing a pale beige suit, was carrying a book about meditation under his arm, was smoking a cigarette, and looked rather agitated. He had a high color, and his behavior was quiet and withdrawn. (During the diagnosis it became clear that his acupuncture color was "lack of white," from a metal imbalance, rather than "red" from a fire imbalance.)

His problem was migraine headaches that felt like a tight band encircling his head. They occurred randomly and unpredictably, and he had been unable to correlate their onset with any dietary habit, weather change, or psychological stress. His migraines generally started in the night, and he was usually awakened by the pain at about 3 a.m. They began to subside by the afternoon. The only accompanying symptom was that his face swelled up around his sinuses, and this trouble might persist for a few days.

His history revealed that, as a baby, he had severe eczema and a tendency to asthma, but he grew out of both of these by the age of seven. He had a happy childhood and had enjoyed school. In college, he had problems in producing written work on time. He said that, although he understood his work well, when he was faced with writing routine essays, his thoughts clogged up, and he felt extremely tired with the effort. In adult life, he became a photographer. He first noticed migraines at the age of 23, but, in the last two years, they had become very frequent and were interfering with his working life. He had tried changing his diet with no success and also tried keeping a diary for three months but had been unable to discover any pattern to his migraines. He was now trying to help himself with meditation. Otherwise, physically, he said he felt "fit as a fiddle," except for a history of constipation since college days and a dry, eczematic skin. During his acupuncture examination, he was found to have a blood pressure of 170/105.

Acupuncture diagnosis showed that his problem came from an imbalance in metal dating from infancy, and, judging by the history of other members of the family and certain other factors, it was congenital. Metal is the element of the lung and colon meridians, which are concerned with bringing in vital *ch'i* energy to the body, mind, and spirit and with eliminating toxins from the body, mind, and spirit.

During his childhood, his body had overcome his problems of asthma and eczema. During his college days, however, the weakness in metal was again sufficient to cause mental and physical constipation; a closed, dry skin; and, a few years later, migraine headaches.

It was decided that, rather than take medication to bring down his blood pressure, which would have the disadvantage of increasing the number of toxins his body had to deal with, he should start acupuncture treatment immediately.

After five treatments, his blood pressure was maintaining at 155/90. He had not had a migraine since the first treatment, but he now came in complaining of very disturbing nightmares. His dreams were chiefly either of airplanes crashing into each other in the sky or of car crashes or of falling out of windows of high buildings. He said that, until the nightmares began, he had been feeling more cheerful and relaxed, but now, perhaps from the effect of the dreams, he was experiencing feelings of vague insecurity by day, also.

His pulse picture revealed that, although the energy in his metal meridians had improved in quality and quantity, the meridians themselves were now unable to deal with the increase in the volume of *ch'i*, and the flow was being dammed up. As the blockage was released, the nightmares stopped. Over a period of a few months, with regular treatment, his bowels started to function normally, his skin gradually became less inert, and he suffered no return of migraine headaches. His blood pressure maintained at 130/85. He comes now for seasonal check-ups.

These two case histories have been chosen because, in acupuncture terms, they both present unusually clearcut cases diagnostically. Most patients will show more of a mixture of elemental imbalances, requiring more detailed analysis to discover the primary cause of their problems.

◎ HELPING ONESELF

To achieve and maintain health we must try to follow the *Tao*, or right way. Most important for maintaining good health is a good diet and exercise regimen, a life of reasonable moderation, and harmony with natural rhythms. "A tranquil conscience fosters *ch'i*," said Mencius, and Chuang Tzu said, "To the mind that is in equilibrium the whole universe surrenders."

◎ PREVENTIVE MEDICINE

Acupuncture may also be practiced as a preventive measure, since the various diagnostic methods signal an imbalance in the meridian system long before this becomes manifested as a symptom. In the past, a Chinese doctor was expected to keep his patients healthy. He was paid as long as the patient was well, but, should the patient fall ill, the doctor had to pay the patient: an early form of medical insurance.

◎ ACUPUNCTURE ANALGESIA

The introduction of Western medicine to China has led to the discovery of another use of the meridian system. This is acupuncture analgesia for use in surgical operations and for pain relief during labor. This method is successful in about 80% of the population. The reason for this is that an anaesthetist can learn a formula of points that are effective for producing analgesia in different areas of the body. If, however, a point in the formula is on a meridian with a congenital, or very severe imbalance, it will not be capable of producing analgesia. It is then necessary to use a different set of points, and it requires someone skilled in traditional acupuncture to determine which meridians can be used.

◎ BAREFOOT DOCTORS

In modern China, also, another use of acupuncture has emerged, particularly in rural areas, in order to deal with the day-to-day health problems of a large population. This is known as "local doctor" or "barefoot doctor" treatment. Barefoot doctors are trained in the use of particular acupuncture points to give first aid for shock, hemorrhage, food poisoning, headache, acute attacks of asthma, structural lesions from injuries, and so on. It is a simplified use of the traditional medical system, but it will, nonetheless, bring dramatic relief in conditions of this kind. The more specialized traditional acupuncturist is called in when a condition arises from chronic imbalance. For instance, a barefoot doctor can use elbow acupuncture points to ease a patient with a pain in the elbow, but, should this trouble arise from a state of general ill health, as in the case of an arthritic elbow, then the effects are only temporary since the cause of the disease has not been corrected. So long as the cause remains, the patient will either re-develop the same symptom or produce a similar symptom elsewhere.

The limited system of barefoot doctor acupuncture has its definite place, but, unfortunately, there are signs that it is traveling to the West and being practiced as though it were a complete system of therapy.

◎ CONCLUSION

Traditional Chinese acupuncture developed out of a cultural tradition of close observation of the dynamic patterns of the macrocosm and microcosm. "The ten thousand things [meaning the cosmos] are there, complete, inside us," said Mencius. This brief and simplified account of the meridian system, with all its implications, is an introduction to the interplay of some of these patterns. It is only individual experience and practice and development of the sensitivity of our perceptions that enables us to understand properly this legacy from the traditional Chinese. In using this system of medicine, we are their humble and grateful inheritors.

REFERENCES ───────────────────────────────

1. Ilza Veith, *Huang-ti Nei-ching Su-wen (The Yellow Emperor's Classic of Internal Medicine* (Berkeley: University of California Press, 1972).
2. *Ibid.*

5

THE STRUCTURAL DIMENSION

DAVID S. WALTHER, D.C.

Mrs. Kelly is somewhat confused as her new doctor finishes his examination. The appointment began routinely enough; she explained to him about the shoulder, which has bothered her on a recurrent basis, even after several types of treatment and medication from her usual physicians. During the first part of the examination, the new doctor felt her shoulder, put it through its range of motion, and tested the muscles of the shoulder for strength. Then the examination began to deviate from a routine one, as the doctor tested muscle strength in other areas of her body. This seemed unusual to Mrs. Kelly, and she should know: she had been to many doctors in recent years for various health problems. She is currently being treated for several conditions. In fact, Mrs. Kelly has so many different problems, she is beginning to feel like a hypochondriac, and her family is becoming impatient with her frequent trips to various physicians. In reaction, Mrs. Kelly has begun minimizing her conditions and does not discuss anything other than her shoulder complaint with this new doctor.

At the conclusion of the examination, the doctor says, "Your shoulder problem is a result of your foot not functioning properly, but I see some other interesting factors also. Do you have burning on urination or problems with incontinence?" Now Mrs. Kelly becomes even more mystified. She admits that she is currently on medication for a bladder infection. How did the doctor know, since he did not have a urinalysis done? "Do you also have problems with digestive gas, muscle or menstrual cramping, or difficulty in getting to sleep?" Again, Mrs. Kelly admits to muscle cramps in her legs, severe menstrual cramping, and digestive gas. The questioning continues, with the new doctor identifying most of the conditions Mrs. Kelly is being treated for by other doctors. What's more, he picks up conditions she is not being treated for: fatigue, depression, and periods of inward shaking and dizziness. Mrs. Kelly had sought the services of a "musculoskeletal" doctor for the relief of some joint pain, and he ended up discussing with her conditions for which she was being treated by four different doctors—one of them a psychiatrist.

What is different about this doctor's examination from those routinely done? To answer this question, it is important that we discuss some of the interactions of body functions and also the interactions of therapeutic approaches.

◎ THE TRIAD OF HEALTH

Various physicians and others involved with restoring health approach a problem from one or more of three basic directions—*struc-*

tural, chemical, or *mental*. These three aspects have become known as the triad of health[1] (Figure 5–1). The triad represents the causes of health problems, and it represents three different approaches to restoring health. Taking one aspect of the triad of health at a time, we can easily observe how health problems develop from a disturbance of that factor and how doctors and others approach the restoration of health through a particular side of the triad. What should be an equilateral triangle, however, often becomes distorted. Too great an emphasis on any one side of the triad may very well limit an individual's opportunity to regain the highest plateau of health.

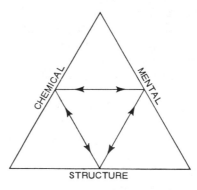

Figure 5–1.   The Triad of Health.

Disturbance in *structure* can influence health in many ways. An abnormal structural balance may cause joint problems, organ encroachment, respiratory disturbance, or muscular strain. Structural distortions also cause impingement upon nerves, which will disturb the function of whatever organ, gland or structure is supplied by that nerve. Many practitioners are involved in improving health by attention to structure. Chiropractors are the largest organized group specifically directing attention to structure to improve health from a natural standpoint. Another system is rolfing,[2] which works to restore structural balance by deep massage of muscles and their fascia. Feldenkrais,[3] Alexander,[4,5] and schools of thought in osteopathy, medicine, and dentistry have approaches to balancing structure by various methods. The orthopedic surgeon uses the allopathic approach to structure.

Health is disturbed from the *chemical* side of the triangle in two ways: an individual may lack nutritional adequacy, or he may be poisoned by chemicals. There are two basic approaches to health included in the chemical side of the triad. The first is treating disease by chemical means, which is primarily the province of the allopathic physician using medications to counteract specific conditions, relieve pain, etc. The second approach is nutrition, practiced by both doctors and laypersons. Within the division of nutritional therapeutics, there is a division in the utilization of nutrition—the allopathic and natural approaches. The allopathic approach uses high dosages of nutrition to counteract a health problem or to cause a specific effect. The natural approach employs correct diet procedures and supplements in dosages found in natural foods.

Finally, the *mental* side of the triad of health includes mental health problems and the spiritual aspect of the individual. Psychologists, psychiatrists, and spiritual leaders all utilize this side of the triad for the improvement of different types of health problems. It is undeniable that an individual's attitude and mental environment have a great bearing on many types of health problems. The psychologist and spiritual counselor provide the natural approach to the improvement of this side of the triad, while the psychiatrist expends an allopathic effort.

Interplay of Triad Factors

Most persons treating health problems are concerned primarily with one side of the triad. However, since there is an interplay between all three sides, there is an effort to affect the other sides by the doctor's specialty. Several examples can illustrate this fact.

Structure Affecting Chemical and Mental. Chiropractors working only with structure regularly influence the endocrine system by correcting distortions that irritate nerves affecting the adrenal medulla. The adrenal medulla secretes hormones and also influences balance of the sympathetic/parasympathetic nervous system, which controls many organs and other glands. Improvement here influences the chemical side of the triad of health.

Alexander's structural approach has also yielded a significant improvement in the mental activity of an individual and demonstrated effective results in many types of psychological problems.

Chemical Affecting Structure and Mental. Allopathic practitioners using the chemical side of the triad influence structure with muscle relaxants and analgesics for the relief of pain. The nutritionist has many different programs of nutritional support for relieving musculoskeletal pain. The problem may be a calcium deficiency, for example, causing muscle cramping. As will be seen later, various nutritional deficiencies can cause actual structural imbalance. The mental side of the triad is approached by those interested in chemistry through tranquilizers, antidepressants, and nutritional products such as niacin and niacinamide.

Mental Affecting Chemical and Structure. It is well known that emotional tension can cause bracing of muscles leading to headaches, jaw pain, pain across the shoulders, etc. Releasing these tensions by various psychological approaches is necessary to bring the structural problem under control. The chemical side of the triad is often influenced by those working with mental processes by returning balance to the autonomic nervous system. This imbalance causes health problems related to organs and glands. The overacid stomach comes to mind as an example of chemical imbalance from emotional stress. This imbalance is often treated through the mental side of the triad of health.

The best approach to evaluate the cause of an individual's health problem is to be well-versed in all three sides of the triad of health, for an involvement of any side can be the result of a problem on another side. In fact, most people who have chronic health problems have involvements on all three sides of the triad. It is the purpose of this chapter to focus on the structural aspect, primarily the musculoskeletal subsystem, and to describe how muscle testing evaluates this dimension of the human being.

INTERPLAY OF BODY SYSTEMS

The interplay present in the triad of health is also present among the systems of the body. A symptomatic problem may not have developed in the system where the patient recognizes it. Decreased blood flow may be apparent because it shows up in the musculoskeletal system as cramps or weakness or in the nervous system as numbness or tingling. Digestive dysfunction may cause poor absorption of calcium, which would be recognized by the musculoskeletal system as cramping and by the nervous system as insomnia or irritability. Kidney involvement can lead to a build-up of uric acid, manifesting itself in the musculoskeletal system as gouty arthritis. The list of one system causing symptoms in another could go on indefinitely because of the interdependence within the body. Most of the examples would be more complicated than those cited here.

The triad of health represents one type of interplay, while the interaction of the systems of the body represents another; both are extremely important in dealing with health problems. Unfortunately, these interactions have not been given the attention they deserve. Probably the major reason they have been overlooked is because of the large volume of knowledge present in today's scientific approach. Doctors have tended to specialize to a high degree. Many investigations designed to find the cause of health problems are limited to a specific system, organ, or structure. As a result, some obvious factor in the condition is recognized, but it is not the basic underlying cause, which may be in another system or from another side of the triad of health. In recent years, there has been a new wave of investigation in human physiology which emphasizes that the body works as an organized, total entity. The term "holistic" has been applied to this health evaluation, which includes all aspects of the triad of health, as well as the integration of the systems in the body.

At first, it may seem there would be great difficulty in evaluating all potential causes and therapeutic approaches while, at the same time, considering the integration of all the systems of the body. Fortunately, this is not the case. The basic fact that the body is totally integrated can be utilized to diagnostic advantage. All systems of the body are interacting continuously with other systems. The musculoskeletal system is of particular interest here because it can be evaluated relatively easily by manual muscle testing. Testing muscles for strength has been a part of neurologic evaluation for many years. Many neurologic and orthopedic texts cover muscle testing for specific nerves. There are texts[6,7] devoted primarily to muscle testing. In 1964, Goodheart[8] began using muscle testing to evaluate patients for structural balance and movement capabilities in his chiropractic practice. The system developed into what is called "applied kinesiology."

Applied kinesiology is the use of muscle testing to evaluate body function and the cause of health problems from a truly holistic standpoint. It uses muscle testing as a diagnostic procedure, evaluating the integration of all of the systems of the body, the influences of the triad of health, and the therapeutic approach best for correction of a health problem. Often, the therapeutic approach is one which eliminates the cause of the problem so that the body can return itself to a state of health. The examination procedures in applied kinesiology are applicable to all disciplines of the healing arts. They are presently used by some members of all professions as discussed earlier with the triad of health.

Shortly after Goodheart began the use of muscle testing, he recognized that many therapeutic approaches previously used affected muscle strength. He also observed a common association of specific muscular weakness with specific organ or gland dysfunction. As more and more therapeutic approaches were found to return muscular strength to normal, the association between muscle function and organ or gland involvement grew stronger, adding to the utilization of muscle evaluation as a diagnostic tool. Looking briefly at some of these interactions will aid in comprehending how the musculoskeletal system is integrated with other systems of the body and provide an idea of how to monitor various functions. If there is dysfunction, this will help in determining what therapeutic approach may be of value.

Musculoskeletal/Nervous System Interaction

The first interaction to be discussed—and probably the easiest to understand—is that of the musculoskeletal with the nervous system. The nervous system is responsible for contraction and organization of the muscular system. This can easily be demonstrated in a normally functioning individual. When a person is walking, there should be subconscious organization of muscle contraction and relaxation in the gait mechanism. Two muscle groups are excellent examples of this activity. During walking, there should be alternate contraction and relaxation of the muscles of the shoulder, which move the arm forward and backward. As the leg goes forward, the muscles in front of the opposite shoulder should slightly contract, bringing the arm forward. At the same time, the muscles in the back of the shoulder should relax, allowing the forward motion. A demonstration of this organization can be accomplished by testing a normal subject in a balanced, standing position (Figure 5–2). A normal subject is one who does not have headaches, neck discomfort, low back pain, legs that get tired when standing, etc.

The flexors (forward movers) and extensors (backward movers) of the shoulder should have approximately equal strength, with both groups being strong, when tested in the balanced standing position. If the subject passes this test, have the individual step forward with the right leg (Figure 5–3). The knee and ankle should be bent in as close to a standard stepping position as possible. Most of the weight will be carried on that leg. The left leg will be trailing with the knee, ankle, and toes flexed and will be only slightly weight bearing. This simulates the stance of walking on the right leg, with the left leg preparing to go into the swing phase. In this position, the extensor muscles of the right shoulder will test weak, while the flexor muscles will test strong. On the left side, the flexor muscles will test weak, and the extensor muscles will test strong. This is the normal activity of facilitation and inhibition of the muscles that alternately turns them on

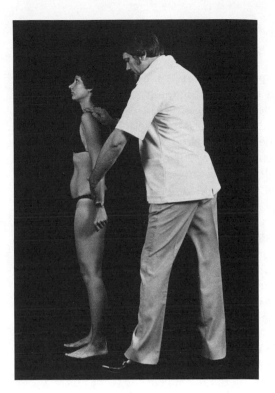

Figure 5–2. Shoulder flexors being tested as a group in a neutral standing position.

Figure 5–3. Shoulder flexors being tested in a simulated gait position. Normal activity is for inhibition of the muscles in this position.

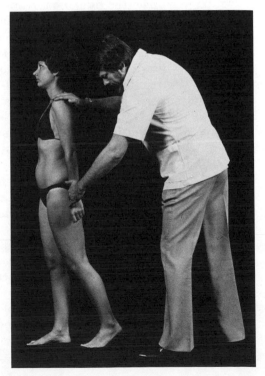

and off during walking. The activity takes place because the nerve endings (proprioceptors) in the joints, ligaments, tendons, and muscles of the feet and legs send information to the central nervous system for organization, ultimately sending instructions to the shoulder flexors and extensors for the activity which should take place at this phase of the gait mechanism. This organization is necessary for the shoulder to function normally. If these muscles are not turning on and off at the appropriate times, tension, fatigue, and achiness will develop in the shoulder. If this persists long enough, bursitis or some other dysfunction of the shoulder will result.

Throughout the body, signals exist for the organization and integration of body function. For various reasons, errors in signaling can develop that are detrimental to body function. In the early stages of the improper signaling, the health problem is functional; that is, there is not pathologic destruction. Ultimately, from continued dysfunction, pathology can result. Whatmore and Kohli[9] refer to this improper signaling as dysponesis.

The demonstration can be extended to illustrate improper signaling by artificially creating a misalignment of the bones of the foot. Two pencils, one placed under the big toe side of the foot and the other under the little toe side, will temporarily cause a dropped metatarsal arch, one of the three arches of the foot. In nearly all normally functioning individuals, this causes confusion in the nervous system. The predictable inhibition and facilitation of the shoulder muscles will no longer take place. When the bones of the foot are misaligned, whether from the experiment just illustrated or from an injury to the foot, the nerve endings are stimulated improperly. The doctor mentioned at the beginning of this article, examining Mrs. Kelly's shoulder, found an imbalance of muscle function there. Evaluating muscles throughout the body, he found that there was a misalignment of one of the bones of the foot, causing the structural imbalance in the shoulder. The previous treatment to her shoulder had no lasting effect because the basic underlying cause of the problem had not been found.

The shoulder is just one example of the consequences of poor foot function. The muscles that support the spinal column, pelvis, knees, and the rest of the skeleton can potentially be out of balance, causing structural distortion and consequent health problems. Spinal column imbalance is significant because spinal nerves can be irritated, affecting organs, glands, or structures throughout the body. It is not uncommon in applied kinesiology to find that headaches, low back pain, and various organ or gland dysfunctions are caused by a foot that has been injured, perhaps even years previously.

The joints and their associated nerve endings (proprioceptors) can be evaluated throughout the body with applied kinesiology techniques. One of these is "challenge" of the articulation. This refers to pushing the joint in various directions and then testing a muscle to determine any change in strength. Under normal conditions, there are specific reactions of various muscles to stimulation of the joint by the challenge mechanism. When the joint is functioning abnormally, there will be lack of normal response of the muscles as observed by the testing procedure. The challenge mechanism not only tells where an involvement is, it also gives information regarding how to manipulate the joint back to normal position. After this is accomplished, the challenge test will no longer show a problem.

The challenge mechanism can be used on any joint of the body. It is frequently used to evaluate for vertebral misalignments or fixations that cause irritations on spinal nerves. The vertebra is extremely important because dysfunction of the spinal nerve can cause organ, gland, muscle, and various tissue problems.

Muscle/Proprioceptor Interaction

Another interaction between the muscular and nervous systems occurs at the proprioceptors of the muscles. Muscles have nerve receptors called neuromuscular spindle cells and Golgi tendon organs, which are located within a muscle or tendon. The purpose of these receptors is to help control the muscle with which they are associated, giving position sense to the body and providing communication with other muscles. Sometimes, when a receptor is injured, it causes the muscle that it resides in to be weak or hypertonic. This, of course, causes a problem with this aspect of the musculoskeletal system, which may manifest as joint pain, structural imbalance, etc. Another type of dysfunction from the muscle proprioceptor is the "reactive muscle." In this situation, a muscle becomes temporarily weak immediately following another muscle's contraction. This happens when incorrect signals go to the secondary muscle because of false information coming from the primary muscle's proprioceptor. Reactive muscles are often found in athletes. In fact, an injury to an athlete can set the stage for more severe problems at a later time. The primary injury, incurred weeks before, can cause a secondary muscle to weaken after specific types of movement. The muscle that weakens may be a knee-supporting one which gives out on an athlete as he is making a quick turn, as often occurs in football and in other sports activities.

Jim's case is typical of a reactive muscle. In football practice, he was hit very hard in the thigh. The quadriceps muscle was swollen and extremely painful, but it did not seem to be injured seriously. The

muscle was packed in ice and treated by massage and other physio-
therapy measures. Unknown at the time, one of the neuromuscular
spindle cells located in the belly of the muscle had been injured and
was over-reacting to quadriceps contraction. If the muscles of Jim's
legs had been tested, it would have been found that another muscle in
his thigh, the sartorius muscle, weakened significantly when tested
immediately after a quadriceps contraction. The reason for this was
the over-reactivity of the neuromuscular spindle cell sending improper signals to the sartorius, causing it to be temporarily inhibited. A
week later, all seemed back to normal. Jim returned to the football
field. When he ran and cut quickly to receive a pass, his leg simply
gave out under him. A torn cartilage resulted, and surgery was necessary for correction. Reviewing movies of the incident later revealed
no apparent reason for Jim's knee to give out. Analysis of the situation, however, revealed that the sartorius weakened immediately
after the quadriceps contraction from running. The sartorius, a medial knee stabilizer, was simply not able to give the necessary aid to
the ligaments in their knee-stabilizing function.

The procedures used in applied kinesiology to return proprioceptors to normal function by manipulation of either the muscle or an
articulation were developed only after a system of diagnosis revealed
the dysfunction to be present. By stimulating various proprioceptors
and then testing muscles to see the effect of the stimulation on them,
much has been learned about the activity of the proprioceptive system. There has already been significant charting of proprioceptor activities in standard physiology research, yet muscle testing techniques are revealing further uncharted activity taking place.

Muscle/Gland Interaction

The nervous system is a very important link in the association between muscle and organ or gland function. When improper nerve activity adversely influences an organ or gland, it can be observed by
testing a specific muscle or muscles associated with that organ or
gland. The muscle will usually be weak, but it could be hypertonic.
The association between muscles and organs and glands was observed
by Goodheart early in applied kinesiology. As additional therapeutic
measures were introduced, the evidence of the association was supported. When normal nerve control returns to the organ or gland, the
muscle also returns to normal strength, thus indicating that correction has been obtained.

Muscle/Meridian System Interaction

A body system recently introduced on a broad scale to the Western world is that of the meridians. Acupuncture is a therapeutic approach for balancing the energy in the meridians of the body. It has been used for thousands of years in oriental countries. The association of muscle strength with organ or gland function in applied kinesiology was enhanced as meridian system balance was found to correlate with muscle test findings.

There are 12 bilateral meridians in the body which the Chinese believe carry the life force, called *ch'i*. These meridians are associated with specific organs and functions of the body. The ten associated with organs of the body are lung, colon, stomach, spleen, heart, small intestine, bladder, kidney, gall bladder, and liver. The two meridians associated with function are the three-heater and circulation-sex. The meridians are evaluated in classic acupuncture for balance of energy. Ideally, the meridians have a good level of energy balanced equally among them. The classic acupuncturist evaluates for an imbalance of the energy pattern of the meridian system, to which he attributes the cause of disease. When imbalance is found, the acupuncturist stimulates various acupuncture points with a needle or through other methods to return balance to the system.

The newly acquired knowledge of the meridian system correlates with muscular weaknesses and hypertonicity found in applied kinesiology muscle testing. It has been discovered that, when a muscle is weak, it can sometimes be strengthened by stimulating the classic acupuncture tonification point for a certain meridian. If the muscle is hypertonic, stimulating the sedation point of the same meridian will bring the muscle back to normal. The interesting correlation is that the meridian which affects a specific muscle also affects the organ or gland with which applied kinesiology had independently correlated the muscle. For example, when an individual has a chest cold or some other involvement with the lung, there will be a weakness or hypertonicity of the deltoid muscle. The meridian that influences deltoid strength or weakness is the lung meridian. This same parallel is present throughout the systems. It was necessary to discover the meridian association for certain muscles, organs, and glands, as there is no meridian specifically correlated with them in classic acupuncture. An example of this is the adrenal gland, which was found to correlate with the circulation-sex meridian.

As mentioned, there are several methods in classical acupuncture for evaluating the energy pattern of the meridian system. These diagnostic methods have been greatly enhanced by the utilization of manual muscle testing to evaluate meridian patterns. Not only can muscle strength indicate when a meridian is out of balance, it also can determine what therapeutic approach is correct for returning the system to balance. This is accomplished by stimulating a potentially appropriate meridian point (or using some other therapeutic method) and observing whether the muscle returns to normal strength. If it does, the therapeutic trial was an effective measure; if not, another approach is obviously needed. With this method of evaluation, many new therapeutic approaches have been found for balancing the meridian system. Some of these do not utilize traditional methods of acupuncture treatment. This will be discussed later as we look at the total integration of body function.

Here is an example of the muscle/meridian interaction applied to a diagnosis of a health problem. Ms. Brown, who had been receiving maintenance health care in our clinic for several years, came in one day with severe abdominal pain. Examination revealed an obvious gall bladder attack, but the curious factor was that gall bladder problems—or for that matter, digestive problems of any type—were not characteristic of this individual. She originally came to the office for treatment of low back pain and decided to use a maintenance approach to health. She had experienced no major health problems for several years. Upon questioning her regarding dietary indiscretions, etc., no positive response was elicited. The muscle associated with the gall bladder is the popliteus, a small muscle behind the knee. It tested very weak, and examination procedures were begun to find which energy pattern, nerve involvement, etc., would cause it to strengthen. Stimulating the tonification point on the gall bladder meridian caused strength to return immediately to the popliteus muscle.

Now comes the question, why was the gall bladder meridian deficient of energy? The sections of the body through which the gall bladder meridian runs were examined, and a small amount of swelling was noted on the outside of the ankle. When Ms. Brown was asked about this, she said, "Oh, yes, I twisted my ankle a little last night when I was walking in the dark and stepped on a rock." The severe pain of the gall bladder attack was diminished within minutes after massaging the swollen area and utilizing very light manipulation to the ankle. This returned normal balance to the gall bladder meridian, and within a half an hour, pain in the abdominal area was totally gone. Ms. Brown's original pain was severe enough that most people would have sought hospital emergency room treatment. The total understanding of the cause of the problem provided a direct method of giving her relief.

Muscle/Reflex Interaction

Reflex treatments, developed many years before applied kinesiology, have become valuable therapeutic tools within its framework. Two of these reflex treatments were developed by Chapman and Bennett, individuals with astute powers of observation and inquisitive natures. Neither of these modalities became very popular, probably because of the lack, at that time, of an objective diagnostic system to validate their use. The development of muscle testing as an evaluation system has made their utilization effective for various types of health problems.

Chapman,[10] an osteopath, developed Chapman's reflex treatments in the 1930s. He claimed that the reflexes influenced lymphatic drainage from various organs and glands. In his studies, he associated different locations as reflexing with various organs, glands, and types of functions of the body. Most of these reflexes are located on the anterior chest and along the spinal column. The active reflex can be palpated (examined by touch) and is usually very tender to the patient. Digital stimulation of an active reflex causes enhancement of the organ or gland function. This is especially true in specific conditions associated with significant lymphatic drainage problems, such as sinusitis, colitis, involvements of the small intestine, etc. The reflex for the lung will consistently be active when an individual has a chest cold or other lung involvement. There will also be weakness of the lung-associated deltoid muscle. Stimulation of the reflex will improve lymphatic drainage of the lungs and immediately strengthen the deltoid muscle. In applied kinesiology, these reflexes are called "neurolymphatic reflexes."

Bennett,[11] a chiropractor, developed a body of reflex treatments in the 1930s which, he claimed, influence the vascular system. These reflexes are located around the body and also correlate with various types of dysfunction and with organs and glands. Again, the correlation of these reflexes fits in with the muscle, organ, and gland association observed in applied kinesiology. The reflexes are treated with a light, tugging, digital touch that produces a pulsation observable to the doctor. The influence of these reflexes on the body can be observed by biofeedback methods, showing an increase in temperatures to various body parts. The treatment of the reflex will immediately strengthen a previously weak muscle that is associated with both the reflex point and its organ or gland. Again, muscle testing gives a diagnostic capability to the reflex system. In applied kinesiology, these reflex points are known as "neurovascular reflexes."

The association between the muscles and organs or glands has become quite solidly defined in applied kinesiology. As more knowledge has been gained, there have been few modifications necessary to Goodheart's original observations. A study was performed at the Anglo-European College of Chiropractic[12] to evaluate the muscle-organ association. An organ was irritated, and the muscle associated with that organ was tested with a spring scale. Then a control muscle was tested. Four organ muscle associations were evaluated: the eye, ear, stomach, and lung. The stomach was irritated by placing cold water into it; the eye with chlorinated water; the ear with sound of a controlled frequency and decibel rate; and the lung with cigarette smoke. In all cases, the associated muscle weakened significantly after the irritation. The control muscle also weakened, but to a much lesser degree. The control muscle weakening parallels the applied kinesiology finding that general muscles of the body weaken when an insult is placed into the nervous system or other controlling factor of the body.

Muscle/Nutritional Interaction

The use of manual muscle testing can be very dramatic in evaluating the nutritional needs of the body. Adverse chemicals will cause a weakening of muscles. These chemicals may be found in the environment, the food supply, or even in intended therapeutic approaches. Adverse chemicals, when placed in the mouth or inhaled, cause any muscle of the body to weaken. There is a more significant weakening of the muscle associated with the organ or gland which the chemical has most affinity to influence. For example, a liver-damaging chemical, such as carbon tetrachloride, will influence the liver-associated muscle—the pectoralis major, sternal division—more than other muscles. When sugar is placed in the mouth of an individual with diabetes or hyperinsulinism, there will be a greater weakening in the latissimus dorsi, associated with the pancreas, than in other muscles of the body.

The association between muscles, organs, and glands continues in the evaluation of nutritional support to various types of function. Nutritional products tend to influence more significantly muscles that have an organ or gland association which correlates with the nutrient being tested. For example, vitamin A supports the pectoralis major, sternal division muscle, which is associated with the liver, while vitamin E tends to influence muscles associated with the reproductive system.

When nutrients are tested with applied kinesiology, they should be chewed and placed under the tongue while the muscle is evaluated.

At times there appears to be some influence on muscular strength when an individual simply holds a nutritional product in the hand or when the product is placed on the body. As many studies have shown, however, under blind conditions, when the examiner performing the muscle test does not know which nutrient has been given nor which route of administration used, hand or body placement of the nutrient turns out to be inaccurate and non-reproducible. It is unfortunate that this inconsistent method is being used by some practitioners, for the oral method is simple and accurate.

While there is significant value in using muscle testing to evaluate nutrition and adverse chemical effects to the body, it is important that the procedure be done in an accurate manner. There has been considerable misuse of manual muscle testing in evaluating nutrition. To help understand this abuse, it is necessary to discuss some of the techniques of testing muscle strength.

APPLIED KINESIOLOGY TECHNIQUES

Many practitioners have contributed to the procedures used in manual muscle testing. There are texts available specifically on manual muscle testing[13, 14] and many orthopedic textbooks have it listed as a system of evaluating nerve function. Manual muscle testing is a precision tool requiring a high degree of knowledge of anatomy and considerable artistry in the application of that knowledge to the testing procedure. It is a system that requires much practice and instruction from qualified teachers.

The body is built in such a way that, for nearly all joint motions, there are numerous muscles contributing to the activity. Manual muscle testing requires knowledge of which muscle is the prime mover in specific motions and which are synergists or helpers. The muscle test begins with a position designed to place the prime mover into its greatest advantage for the testing activity, while the synergists are at the greatest possible disadvantage. During the testing procedure, the examiner must apply a vector of force specifically designed to test the prime mover. He must use his knowledge of what synergists will attempt to take over if the prime mover is weak. Furthermore, many testing procedures rely on fixation of specific body parts by adequate action of the patient's "fixator" muscles. All these considerations must be applied as the examiner initiates his test. The testing force must be applied with a specific speed and vector and at the correct point of contact (Figure 5–4).

Careful monitoring for slight changes of patient position is nec-

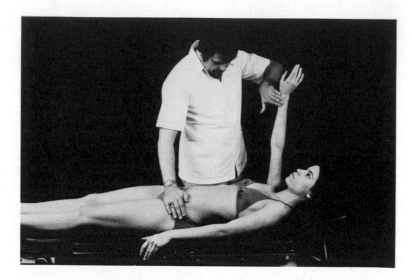

Figure 5–4. Correct testing procedure for the pectoralis major—sternal division. Note the examiner stabilizing at the hip with his right hand while the elbow is kept in extension. A non-overpowering force is being used at the examiner's left-hand fingertips.

essary, as they may indicate a subconscious effort to recruit synergist activity. The patient's body will attempt to be strong during the testing procedure. Since there are usually several muscles that have synergistic capabilities to the prime mover being tested, very slight changes of patient position, etc., can make the muscle appear to be strong when it is not. The examiner must also know what factors change muscle strength because, again, the patient's body will attempt to maneuver its energy patterns to supplement weak areas. These factors of the science and art of muscle testing are not presented to make manual muscle testing look complicated; it is not. It simply requires adequate anatomical knowledge, mastery of the principles of the test, and developed art in testing which comes only from practice.

General group muscle testing should not be used for evaluating nutrition or organ-muscle association because there are too many variables present. Many practitioners of applied kinesiology have done studies on general muscle testing, such as an arm pull-down test, and found poor reproducibility of the quasi-testing procedure (Figure 5–5). The only time groups of muscle tests should be used is when they are part of a specific function, such as the shoulder flexors

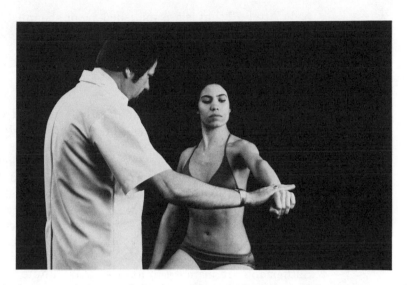

Figure 5–5. The arm pull-down test has considerable variables and is not easily reproduced for accuracy.

or the extensors of the gait motion illustrated earlier in this chapter. Unfortunately, much muscle testing is done to evaluate health problems and the influences of nutrition on the body without adequate background in the science and art of the procedures involved. This is probably due to the fact that there has been a lot of publicity in books and magazines for the lay public on the use of muscle testing to evaluate the various factors that influence health. The only reason this writer is opposed to this type of naive general use of the technique is because of the considerable amount of personally observed, inaccurate muscle testing being done. This uninformed use of the procedures can give erroneous information about the effects of the various items being tested on the body. Many times, the errors come from operator prejudice. For example, some individuals who have great prejudice against white sugar will find evidence of muscular weakness in everyone who puts white sugar in their mouth or holds it in their hand. This global result, of course, is inaccurate. Certain metabolic types can tolerate white sugar with no adverse effects to the body.

Muscle testing is a viable tool for the evaluation of body function. However, it is no better than the examiner's capabilities. Any individual utilizing muscle testing to evaluate body function should have a good knowledge of the body's anatomy, of the physiology of the interactions of muscular function, and of the general physiology of the body. After all that is accomplished, he or she must be willing to dedicate the hundreds of hours necessary to perfect the art of muscle testing under the direction of a qualified instructor.

Cranial Respiration/Muscle Correlation

Another functional system that can be evaluated very efficiently by applied kinesiology is the cranial primary respiratory system, or motion between the bones of the skull. This system is not as well known in the healing arts as others, even though knowledge of it has been available for many years. Sutherland[15] published findings of his research in cranial articular mobility that dated back to 1899. With astute observation of the cranial structure and very careful palpatory investigation, he devised an apparatus to restrict movement of his own skull. The restricted movement of the skull caused specific types of neurological dysfunction. The motions of the skull described by Sutherland are primary in nature. This minute motion is necessary for normal cerebrospinal fluid function, cranial nerve activity, and prevention of disturbances that can be caused by lack of normal function in this area. Although the primary cranial respiratory mechanism is independent of diaphragmatic breathing, it is influenced by it.

Many times, muscular weakness is present because of a cranial fault; that is, a section of the cranial respiratory mechanism is not moving correctly. This lack of normal motion usually develops as a result of trauma to the skull or imbalanced muscular force affecting the skull. Many cranial faults develop from birth trauma. If the problem is not corrected, the skull will ossify in a structurally unsound position. The birth trauma may be the beginning of a lifetime of health problems. The earlier in life these are corrected, the better the correction will be and the greater the health improvement.

When a muscle is weak as a result of a cranial fault, it can be strengthened if the subject takes and holds a specific phase of diaphragmatic respiration. When this is done, the muscle immediately becomes strong and remains that way as long as that phase of respiration is held. Because the skull moves in a specific manner with diaphragmatic respiration, this gives diagnostic information as to which way the cranium should be manipulated in order to unlock it and return normal motion.

Evaluating the cranial mechanism by observing how muscles change strength at different phases of respiration and by using the challenge mechanism described earlier, makes the analysis of cranial faults easy and accurate. Challenge is utilized by mild pressure applied to various areas of the skull. These pressures will not influence muscle strength if there is no cranial fault present at that area. If there is one, there will be a temporary weakening of a muscle that will last long enough for the examiner to observe the change. The challenge and diaphragmatic respiratory influences on the cranium give specific information of how to correct the body. The system is a method of testing for skull motion to determine what corrections may be necessary.

◎ OTHER THERAPIES

Many therapeutic approaches have been developed, frequently on an empiric basis, which appear to have no scientific basis for effectiveness in treating health problems. Yet the various systems are developing followings because of apparent results where orthodox approaches have failed. Evaluation of body function through the structural dimension with applied kinesiology techniques has provided an explanation of the results of some of these therapeutic approaches. Foot reflexology is a case in point.

Foot Reflexology

Most foot reflexologists locate the sinus reflex along the bottom surface of the toes. This is in the area of the tendons of the flexor digitorum longus muscle. The muscle is located in the lower leg, with its tendons extending into the foot to attach to the distal portion of the toes. The proprioceptors located in these tendons associate with the muscles that flex the neck and head forward. This can be seen by stimulating these proprioceptors of the flexor digitorum longus muscle and then observing the inhibition or weakening of the muscles in the neck on manual muscle testing. These are the muscles associated with the sinuses in applied kinesiology. Some type of dysfunction in the foot (usually a tarsal tunnel syndrome) can cause improper weight-bearing and imbalance of the foot muscles. This causes stimulation to the proprioceptors in the toes which is not consistent with the actual function of the foot. The resulting neurologic confusion will cause weakness of the neck flexor muscles. Prolonged dysfunction of these neck muscles will ultimately affect the sinuses by activation of the sinus neurolymphatic or neurovascular reflexes, upper cervical spinal subluxations, or involvement with the cranial primary respiratory mechanism. Any or all of these factors can cause sinus problems.

It may seem strange to an individual who does not consider the body from a holistic viewpoint to think sinus problems can come from foot dysfunction. The fact remains that the body is a totally integrated structure, and improper stimulation of nerves, regardless of the origin, can create remote health problems. The foot is a significant source of improper nerve impulses that enter into the neuronal pools and create confusion at any place in the body.

The foot reflex generally described for large intestine involvements is in the general location of a small bone in the foot called the cuboid. Misalignment of this bone from an injury often causes weakness in the tensor fascia lata muscle of the thigh, associated in applied kinesiology with the large intestine. The mechanism of the foot misalignment causing weakness in the tensor fascia lata correlates with the physiologic reflex called the magnet reflex. Its purpose is to supply information to the muscles that control lateral sway of the body to contract or relax when pressure is applied to the side or medial aspect of the foot, as happens when the body begins to sway to the side. This is part of the balance mechanism of which the tensor fascia lata muscle is a part. Constant improper function of the muscle as a result of incorrect information coming from the foot will cause activation of some or all of the many physiologic associations of this muscle. The mechanism is similar to that described above for the sinuses. It could be an activation of a neurolymphatic or neurovascular reflex, misalignments in the spinal column, or an imbalance of the large intestine meridian. Stimulation of the large intestine reflex by the foot reflexologist can improve the tensor fascia lata muscle function, removing its adverse influence over the numerous factors that correlate it with the large intestine. Thus, a simple stimulation of a point in the foot can improve large intestine function.

Foot reflexology can sometimes correct foot problems. When actual correction is obtained, it is by luck and not by designed effect. Unfortunately, if the foot problem is only influenced by the foot reflexologist's treatment and not corrected, the symptomatic improvement of the sinus or colon conditions illustrated will only be temporary. The actual dysfunction of the foot must be corrected for permanent results. In the illustrations given, the foot is the primary area of involvement. It causes remote symptoms by influencing some type of control mechanism or energy pattern.

If the foot involvement has just recently occurred, as in the example of Ms. Brown's gall bladder attack, the correction is immediate. There is the possibility in a chronic condition, on the other hand, that, in addition to correcting the foot dysfunction, it may be necessary to attend to the secondary factors. In other words, a prolonged problem with the sinus or large intestine may require nutritional support or localized treatment to the muscle or organ. If the foot is ignored and treatment is given only to the secondary area, it will probably be effective but not lasting. After treatment is discontinued or stress returns to the organ or secondary structure, the symptom associated with the secondary area will return. Treatment to the secondary area is often needed when the condition has become chronic and other sides of the triad of health are involved.

ROLFING

Rolfing is a system of evaluating structural balance and applying therapeutic deep massage to correct disturbed balance. The system has gained a certain amount of popularity, and many claims of improvement of various health problems have come from both therapists and patients using the approach. One of the basic tenets of the system is that a muscle and its fascial cover can get out of balance with each other, thus disturbing function. This appears to be confirmed in applied kinesiology by manual muscle testing, using a specific type of analysis. The procedure is to test a muscle to determine normal strength. If normal strength is present, it can be evaluated for balance between the muscle and fascia by stretching the muscle and fascia and then immediately re-testing the muscle for strength. When the muscle and fascia are not in balance, the second muscle test will reveal a weakening. A deep massage of the muscle and fascia, such as that used in rolfing, will eliminate this positive response.

A most interesting aspect of this therapeutic approach is the change in the organ or gland that is associated with the muscle thus treated. An easy association to observe is that of the teres minor muscle, a shoulder rotating muscle, with the thyroid gland. In hypothyroidism, there is a reduced temperature level in the body.[16] After evaluating for the muscle stretch response and treating it, there will be an immediate rise in temperature as measured by the standard thermometer approach or by thermal biofeedback equipment. The rise in temperature is a consistent finding when deep massage is applied to an involved teres minor muscle; however, it is not present when the same therapeutic approach is used on muscles associated with other organs or glands. It must be understood that not all hypothyroidism is involved with a need for this type of therapeutic approach to the teres minor muscle.

MUSCLE TESTING FOR THE MENTAL ASPECT

Illustrations have been given of how muscle testing can be utilized to evaluate the structural and chemical sides of the triad of health. The mental side is also represented in muscular function as observed by manual muscle testing. Here, too, there is a correlation with the association of various muscles with the different organs and glands of the body. The association is not as clearcut as the chemical and structural factors because emotions tend to affect the entire body.

It is relatively easy with muscle testing to observe an emotional factor that is influencing an individual's health. When an emotional stress is introduced, a previously strong muscle will weaken. If the emotional stress is strong enough, almost any muscle in the body will show the change. The best way to observe an emotional effect on the body is to test a specific aspect. For example, if digestive problems are suspected to be caused by emotional disturbance, the examiner can test the muscles associated with different aspects of digestion, such as the clavicular division of the pectoralis major muscle for the stomach and the tensor fascia lata muscle for the colon. If these muscles test strong, the examination procedure can begin. If the muscles are not strong, the examiner must find and use the appropriate therapeutic approach to strengthen them. The patient is then requested to concentrate on a suspected emotional problem. It may be a situation at work, a marital problem, a delinquent teenage son, or whatever.

As the patient concentrates on a specific emotional problem affecting his health, there will be a weakening of muscles of his body. The weakening will be most dramatic in muscles associated with organs or glands being influenced by the stress. If the individual is having digestive problems correlating primarily with stomach dysfunction, the clavicular division of the pectoralis major muscle will weaken. If hyperperistalsis and subsequent problems are developing in the colon, the tensor fascia lata muscle will weaken most significantly. The same concept can be extended to evaluate other organs and glands, such as the adrenal glands, which are frequently disturbed as a result of emotional stress. This system of evaluation helps to find problems that need a further therapeutic approach (for example, counseling) to recognize and control the problem, or the system can recommend action to alleviate it, such as changing jobs.

Although mental health counseling and spiritual advisement are very important aspects in the holistic approach to health care, it must be recognized that many of the mental problems from which people suffer are caused by dysfunction of basic physiology within the body. Many who have significant depression and are unable to cope with the daily stresses placed upon them by the environment have a blood-sugar-handling dysfunction as the basic underlying cause. During periods of the day, the blood sugar drops to such low levels that the nervous system, both peripheral and central, simply cannot function optimally. Mental confusion develops, and what would ordinarily be a simple problem to handle cannot be managed. If this condition becomes chronic, the sufferer will obviously develop actual emotional stress because he cannot handle the requirements of employment or relate well with the people in his environment. By this stage, counseling may be significantly needed; however, it will not be effective until the basic underlying cause of the sugar-handling problem is eliminated. Then counseling becomes easier and more productive.

Evaluating the interactions of the mental, chemical, and structural sides of the triad of health becomes invaluable in finding the basic cause underlying the psychological complaint. Evaluating only the primary complaint can lead to a lifetime of continuing mental health problems.

No therapeutic approach provides a total answer to health problems. The discussion has been limited to simple interactions between systems of the body. The limitation of the length of this chapter precludes more sophisticated discussion of the interactions within the body. It is specifically because of these interactions that many new therapeutic approaches have been devised and introduced into practice in the framework of applied kinesiology. All individuals dealing with health—especially those dealing with illness—must have knowledge of the interactive nature of total body function and of the approaches to correction of dysfunction. The same type of interaction that has been described for the musculoskeletal system with other systems of the body is present among all systems. The advantage of the musculoskeletal system is that it is easy to evaluate by proper manual muscle testing. The primary rule of diagnosis is that you cannot recognize what you do not know!

REFERENCES

1. David S. Walther, *Applied Kinesiology—The Advanced Approach in Chiropractic* (Pueblo, CO: Systems DC, 1976).
2. Ida P. Rolf, *Rolfing* (Santa Monica, CA: Dennis-Landman, 1977).
3. Moche Feldenkrais, *Awareness Through Movement* (New York: Harper & Row, 1972).
4. F. Matthias Alexander, *Resurrection of the Body*, ed. Edward Maisel (New York: a Delta book, 1969).
5. Wilfred Barlow, *The Alexander Technique* (New York: Alfred A. Knopf, 1973).

6. Lucy L. Daniels, Marian Williams, and Catherine Worthingham, *Muscle Testing*, 2d edition (Philadelphia: W.B. Saunders Co., 1956).

7. Henry O. Kendall, Florence P. Kendall, and Gladys E. Wadsworth, *Muscles—Testing and Function*, 2d edition (Baltimore: Williams and Wilkins Co., 1971).

8. George J. Goodheart, Jr., *Applied Kinesiology Research Manual, 1964–1979* (Detroit: privately published).

9. George B. Whatmore and Daniel R. Kohli, *The Physiopathology and Treatment of Functional Disorders* (New York: Grune and Stratton, Inc., 1974).

10. Frank Chapman, *An Endocrine Interpretation of Chapman's Reflexes*, ed. Charles Owens, (publisher and date unknown).

11. T.J. Bennett, *Dynamics of Correction of Abnormal Function*, ed. Ralph J. Martin, (Sierra Madre, CA: privately published, 1977).

12. S.A. Carpenter, J. Hoffmann, and R. Mendel, "Evaluation of Muscle-Organ Association," *Journal of Clinical Chiropractic*, Vol. II, no. 6, Part I, pp. 22-33; Vol III, no. 1, Part II, pp. 42-60.

13. Kendall, Kendall, and Wadsworth, *loc. cit.*

14. Daniels, Williams, and Worthingham, *loc. cit.*

15. William G. Sutherland, *The Cranial Bowl* (Mancato, MN: Free Press Co., 1939).

16. Broda O. Barnes and Lawrence Dalton, *Hypothyroidism—The Unsuspected Illness* (New York: Thomas Y. Crowell Co., 1976).

6

THE BREATHING DIMENSION

CAROLA H. SPEADS

Breathing means life; not breathing is death. Breathing is one function our body cannot do without. We can survive without limbs, without certain organs, or with sick organs, but we cannot survive without breath. The intake of oxygen and the elimination of carbon dioxide is essential for our existence. Our body in its totality depends on breathing. Our skeleton, our muscles, our circulation, our joints, our organs, our brain—all processes in our body rely on breathing. Respiration is necessary for all parts of our body to fulfill their tasks and to eliminate their waste products. Each cell in our body depends on our breathing in order to function properly.

As our brain depends on oxygen supply, our thinking and creativity depend on breathing. Even our moods depend on the quality of our breathing. They are attuned to it and happen in unison with it. All thinking and feeling is mirrored simultaneously in the way we breathe. In fact, the quality of our breathing influences the quality of our lives; our health, mood, energy, and creativity.

The fact that our bodily functions depend on breathing is generally accepted. But the interdependence of our moods and thinking with breathing and the effects of breathing quality upon our mood, intelligence, and creativity are less generally acknowledged. We all have a wide range of experience with these interrelationships. We have all felt our breathing change markedly in stressful situations, pleasant as well as unpleasant, and we've all noticed it become irregular or maybe even stop at times. Often, a struggle for breath ensues, at times long lasting, until the blissful moment when, finally, a usual way of breathing returns. And who does not remember the forcing of breath when we cried hard as a child: our whole body shook!

Although we tend to repress breathing experiences, they show up clearly in our language: we heave a "sigh of relief"; we listen with "breathless attention." Excitement "takes our breath away," we show an "air of confidence," we "hurry through in the same breath," we "take a breather," and we are "puffed up with pride."

◎ BEING SUPPORTED BY BREATH

Our typical shallow breathing is adequate at rest, but we must breathe deeper and faster when we need more oxygen for heavy physical labor, sports, concentration on an important decision, or for a creative flow of images. Our competence in dealing with other people also depends on our breath. If, in the course of a business meeting, breathing changes for the worse and becomes restrained or irregular, we can realize instantaneously that something is wrong. Perhaps the other person does not understand us or does not mean what he or she proposes and is trying to cheat us. The opposite also holds true. When we find that, during an important interview, our breathing changes for the better—that we draw deep breaths—we know we are in good hands and confronted by someone who means well.

Breathing is an involuntary process. We cannot change it willfully; we can only stimulate it or coax it to change quality. This is done mainly, but not only, by aiming at more efficient exhalations. Fuller inhalations follow automatically. Awareness of ourselves and of our breathing in particular gives the data for such work. By feeling and acknowledging changes in the quality of our breathing when they occur, we can shorten recovery from stress.

A student arrived before a workshop in order to talk to me. He was in despair because someone close to him had died. He had to write a letter and was too disturbed to write. I acknowledged that this was a sad and upsetting event for him, and I understood that he was deeply disturbed. I urged him to stay and work along with us. Through our work, he became aware that his breathing was shallow and that his whole body was tense. He became aware of how he rushed himself from one breath to the next, eliminating the breathing pause and thus forcing too fast a breathing rhythm. He also felt keenly the lack of satisfaction that adequate breathing conveys. By letting his exhalations flow out more freely, his breathing rhythm slowed down. He was no longer compelled to force his breaths in and out. Simultaneously, his tension eased, and he regained normal tone, changing from an almost crouched bodily position to one of upright balance. His hands, which had been cramped into fists, loosened. After the session, he was calmer and could face the difficult situation. He was confident he could find the right words for the letter he had to write.

There is no best way of breathing or one that should prevail at all times. The main feature of our breathing is that it is adjustable. It should function adequately for whatever we are doing or living through and should change its quality according to our immediate needs. When we sit quietly and have a nice chat with a good friend, our breathing is easygoing. When we are applying for a job, or driving in heavy traffic, or overjoyed, or afraid, or furious, our breathing will differ in quality. Running, sleeping, reading—each requires specific kinds of breathing. Different conditions affect us differently and elicit different support from our breathing. We must let our breath adjust appropriately to a given situation.

Breathing reactions do not follow the impact of events on us. They occur simultaneously with the impact, comparable to our getting in front of a mirror, where our picture appears at the same time we get in front of it. The actual changes in breathing are the same for pleasure and distress. Holding our breath, for example, may be caused through quite contrary events—curiosity as well as terror. Our whole person, and that includes our breathing, responds to any change in our individual world.

DISTURBANCES OF BREATHING

The quality of our breathing is disturbed by many elements in our way of life. Crime, war, political unrest, noise and air pollution, sudden general or personal changes too far reaching for easy adjustment, mechanization threatening our sense of value as individuals: these and other stresses of modern life can disturb our breathing.

As an involuntary process, breathing reacts automatically to stress. But, unlike other autonomic functions, breathing is also controlled by the voluntary nervous system. So we can interfere with the breathing process. We interfere with its rhythm by temporarily holding the breath, breathing too fast or too slow, or shortening or prolonging the breathing pause. We can also disturb the basic breathing process by interfering with exhalation or inhalation (often with both)—trying to help instead of letting the breath stream freely at the speed and intensity required by the moment. After the excitement or stress has passed, our voluntary "help" may remain in operation. Our breath is no longer quiet and easy at rest. Rather, it is kept too shallow. And now, fixed in a specific breathing pattern, we can no longer react to new situations with natural, flexible breathing.

Some people recover quickly, almost rebound, to normal as soon as strain eases. Others take long periods to recoup a normal way of breathing and, with that, a normal way of functioning. Many cling to states of disturbed breathing for years, some even for the rest of their lives. Disturbances in other dimensions, such as excess tension, contribute to the inability to recover the normal adjustability of breathing. Inefficient breathing may be enough to keep us alive, but it results in minimum stamina. Most persons with lowered breathing efficiency have little energy, tire easily, and recuperate slowly from illness. Others, in order to bear up, become high strung and overreact to events. Their minds do not work efficiently. They are certainly not the ones to give us great ideas or inventions. Their emotional reactions are usually not appropriate to life challenges.

Some of us suffer greatly from such conditions, and others use them to their advantage. "We all have our peculiarities, and this is mine," a student once said to me. With this excuse, she could get away with almost anything. "I am the nervous type," someone else said. That conviction gave him a reason to decline any task or duty he did not like.

Whenever we have interfered with the functioning of our breathing for any length of time, emergency measures like yawning, heaving, sighing and stretching set in to restore breathing efficiency. Well known to all of us is yawning. It will happen, for instance, when we are bored, a state characterized by our breathing becoming shallower and shallower. Yawning, a violent contraction of the diaphragm, enforces a strong exhalation and inhalation. We have all experienced, often to our embarrassment, that we cannot stop yawning at will; it has to stop by itself. And it does, as soon as the breathing emergency is relieved. While we do not choose to yawn, heave, sigh, or stretch, we must let these reactions loose. Emergency measures are true physical urges that overpower us. They abate gradually as the breathing recovery progresses. By accommodating these urges rather than stifling them, we shorten the time needed for breathing recoveries.

Certain disturbances of emotions show different kinds of breathing. Overexcitement accelerates the breathing rhythm and shortens the breathing pause. Depression is characterized by irregularity of the breathing rhythm, by repeated long pauses followed by sighs, and by isolated, deep, often sighing breaths. Feeling rushed is accompanied by too fast, too shallow breathing, by periods of holding the breath, and by foreshortening the breathing pause or skipping it altogether. Rushing and feeling rushed are particularly detrimental to health and can be easily spotted by paying attention to the breath.

A new student, a bookkeeper, complained that for years she was burdened with too much work. She felt rushed and taken advantage of. When she started to work with me, she had no awareness at all of her breathing. She was unable to feel whether her breath was flowing or whether she held it. She had not an inkling of the quality of her breathing; she was unaware of whether it served her adequately or whether she lacked its support. She was totally estranged from this vital bodily function.

In the first stage of work, she concentrated on feeling that she was breathing. Then, with help, she became aware of the fact that she interfered with her breathing. Eventually, she felt how she interfered. At the same time, she found that her breathing responded favorably to such stimuli as a gentle tapping of her rib cage, prolongation of her exhalations, or slight pressure on the ribs. In time, she discovered that her body tone, her physical endurance under stress, and her stamina depended on the manner of her breathing and that her breath influenced her mood. Her thinking was clearer and her activity more when her breathing supported her properly.

Her main concern was work, so she focused on the relationship between her breathing and how she performed her bookkeeping tasks. She began to interrupt work to take care of her breath when necessary. When she was alone, she tapped herself; when not alone, she opened her mouth just slightly, so as not to draw attention to herself, and let air stream out more freely. She gradually became able to work feeling less pressure. She no longer felt so burdened that she was forced to rush.

Eventually, she was able to work peacefully. Because she did not waste energy and time on inefficient breathing, she now had ample time to do her job. She worked calmly and with easy concentration, not nervously as before. Instead of endlessly checking and re-checking her figures, she felt sure of her work and gained time. There even came an occasional period when she was bored because she had nothing to do. She stressed that absolutely nothing in her job had changed. She had the same number of books to keep and business was the same as before. The only factor that had changed was her breathing.

◎ BREATHING WORK

Breathing therapy assumes the total unity of the human being, and its results show the interrelation of body, mind, and emotions. Breathing work can successfully effect an increase in circulation, normalize tonus (the fundamental tension that exists independent of voluntary action), clarify thinking, and improve mood. In this approach, we experience how our breathing is working during any given moment, feel the ways it may be interfered with, and see what can be done to let it function more effectively.

Though the ways and means by which we are able to interfere with our breathing are generally the same for all of us, each individual uses them in a decidedly unique way. Thus, there are innumerable, slightly different manifestations of interference, and there is an endless variety of poor breathing habits to overcome. We must become aware of how we interfere with our breathing and how we react to life situations that disturb our equilibrium.

Consequently, breathing work should be geared to individual needs. Using fixed exercises is not only boring but also inefficient. Utilizing instead an immense variety of approaches to induce efficient breathing makes results more far-reaching. Procedures are then continually exciting and interesting. Changes in the quality of the breath are achieved through experimentation, not through repetitive and mechanistic exercises. Because breathing is so variable, an infinite number of exercises would be necessary. Besides, we do not exercise a self-regulatory function, such as breathing, like we exercise a muscle. Breathing can only be coaxed to change by using certain beneficial stimuli. Reactions to a stimulus must be allowed to develop as freely as possible and should be felt and studied.

In doing breathing work, we rely on our body sense, our kinesthetic sense, for feedback. This enables us to become aware of ourselves, feel the position of our body in space, and feel the condition of our body. Sensations inform us of the state of our breathing and of our reactions to the experiments. As we progress, we sense with increasing precision how our breathing reacts to particular experiments. We also become aware of innumerable variations in the quality of our breathing.

A few examples of sensations we may become aware of are the flow of air through our nose and mouth, irregularities in rhythm, senses of frustration or satisfaction (such as the feeling of relief when an inhalation finally gets through), and a sense of depth in breathing. A most impressive sense that comes after breathing work is the extremely quiet and effortless way in which our breath can flow. How still we have to perceive this new sense! When we get to this stage, we have achieved a remarkable difference in the quality of our breathing.

As we start a breathing experiment, we should allow whatever time is necessary to let our breathing change. Reacting quickly one day does not mean we will react quickly the next. In breathing work, we must be flexible and let nature work at her own speed.

Check your breathing before you start an experiment. In that way you can notice, compare, and evaluate the breathing differences arrived at through an experiment. Evaluation is vitally important for successful breathing work. The pre-exercise checkup involves answering several questions:

1. "Do I feel anything at all related to my breathing?" At first, it seems no answer is available, but as awareness increases, sensations become more evident.
2. "Where, specifically, do I feel something related to my breathing?" We will notice which areas of our body are involved in breathing and to which areas breathing spreads.
3. "What does my breathing feel like?" What are its characteristics and its quality? It is labored or easy, restricted or full, shallow, rhythmic, weak, or uneven?

In all experiments, it is important to wait until average breathing has re-established itself before repeating the experiment. If we re-stimulate our breathing while still reacting to a previous stimulus, our breathing will become erratic, and we will be extremely uncomfortable for a while.

A good experiment for beginners is to breathe through a straw, as it leads easily to increased inhalation. By letting air stream out freely through the straw, you expel more air than you would ordinarily. The more air goes out, the more air has to come in. Also, since air can get out only through the narrow straw, the diaphragm is forced to relax slowly rather than suddenly; thus, the main breathing muscle is toned up.

Another experiment uses the largest possible passage, a wide open mouth. After doing a checkup on your breathing, feel when exhalations and inhalations occur. Shortly after the start of an ordinary exhalation, open your mouth wide, and let air stream out as freely as possible. The air should flow out of its own accord without the slightest pushing or forcing. In contrast to the straw, you now offer the air a passageway for exhalation as wide as a barn door.

Using the vocal cords in exhalation increases energy and, therefore, helps breathing recuperate from sluggishness. Sound generates body awareness with which to judge the quality of breathing. Humming is valuable and can be varied by adding vowels. Projecting a sibilant "S" horizontally forward and aiming for a long, loud, steady sound results in fuller exhalations. These are followed by deeper inhalations. It is easy to judge whether an "S" sound was steady, strong, quavery, or weak. Hence, was it a good breath or a poor one?

Exhalation on the palm offers a particularly gentle way to increase exhalations and thus induce deeper inhalations. Holding the palm vertically and fairly close to the mouth, let a single exhalation through the mouth waft gently onto the palm while making a soft, barely audible, continuous "haaaa" sound, as in harvest. We breathe in a similar way, only forcefully, to clean eyeglasses or a mirror. But doing the experiment, the breath should stream out of the mouth gently and as much on its own as possible. This soft "haaaa" sound is restful, affecting our breathing by calming it and making it fuller.

During breathing work, we become aware, sometimes quite suddenly, that our rib cage is not elastic enough to accommodate comfortably our now fuller breaths. Our rib cage feels stiff and does not expand as much as our inhalations soon require. It should expand in all directions like a balloon: up, down, forward, and backward. We can experiment with grasping a skinfold or applying pressure to help overcome this curtailing of inhalation. The skinfold should be lifted just barely off the rib cage in a direction away from the center of the body; that is, approximately forward in front, laterally on the sides, and backward from the back. A skinfold is grasped, lifted, and held off its base until a deeper breath gets through. Then it is released. Lift-

ing a skinfold has the same effect as opening a too-tight belt or bras-
siere after having worn it for a good while: we immediately expand
and draw a deep breath of relief as we get free.

Very light pressure—light fingertip pressure applied over the
whole rib cage, on the breastbone, or on and between the ribs—is another means of regaining elasticity in the rib cage. The rib cage fills
up more fully after the applied pressure is released—pressure being
a stimulus. Also, when the rib cage opens up, the diaphragm has then
a wider span and works more efficiently.

Movements, like those in normal daily activities, can also stimulate breathing if we let our breathing adapt without interference.
Breathing would give us adequate support automatically, but most of
us hinder our breath during movements by holding it, pressing on it,
or inhaling willfully instead of letting the breath flow in freely. In so
doing, we rob ourselves of a most effective support for movement and
thus interrupt the process of getting ample oxygen and eliminating
carbon dioxide just at the moment of need. We can also stimulate
breathing by stretching. Or we can try everyday movements or assume postures that passively expand the rib cage, always trying to
feel and let all reactions of our breathing through.

We can use sensing of our breathing, without applying any particular stimulus, to let our breathing recover from strain or to maximize efficiency before embarking on important activities. Physical
and emotional strength will then be at our disposal. This experiment
has three phases.

First, feel the exhalations without interference. (A few helpful
questions to ask here are, "Do my exhalations happen on their own, or
do I interfere with them?" "Do I tamper with the outflow of air by
holding back or pushing out?" "Am I giving my exhalations the full
time they need?") As we become more aware of the ways in which we
disturb our breathing, we disturb it less and less.

Second, simply feel the inhalations. Earlier experience with exhalations makes it easier to attend to inhalation and overcome interference. Gradually, inhalations will function more on their own.

Third, we watch the breathing pause, trying to sense what it is
we do and how we interfere with the self-regulating of the transition
between exhalation and inhalation. As we interfere less with this
transition, the appropriate length of pause re-establishes itself. This
is essential to efficient and satisfying breathing rhythm.

The conscious experience of the rhythm, constancy, and effectiveness—in short, of the support—of our breathing is a wonderfully gratifying experience. Through experiments such as those described, we
recover an ease and fullness of breath that we may not remember feel-

ing before. We experience physical well-being, calmness, and serenity. Our personal attitudes change.

It is an amazing experience to feel how, with the recovery of our breathing, our outlook on life changes. Simple things like a ray of sunshine can now please us. Will we be breathless and overwhelmed or will we have the support of our breathing to withstand onslaughts? The steadfastness we need at times depends on the energy and support given to us by our breath. Our breath is important in coping with the troubles and pleasures life brings. Our greatest help in securing this support is that our breathing has an innate tendency to recover from disturbance. This is, as a student put it recently, ". . . so comforting to experience. In our insecure times when everything is constantly changing there is something that reacts invariably in the same manner . . . something you can always rely on. My breathing reacts at all times positively whenever I give it a chance."

The state of our breathing is decisive for the well-being and well-functioning of our whole person. Taking care of breathing affects us in our totality.

REFERENCES

Carola H. Speads, *Breathing, The ABC's* (New York: Harper & Row, 1978).

7

THE AWARENESS DIMENSION

ROBERT K. HALL, M.D. AND
JAMES THOMAS POPE

An interrelatedness pervades all phenomena. Never are we out of relationship with anything that exists. We can be aware of our bodies because all sensation happens in the body and is translated into information in the central nervous system. We can be aware of our minds because thoughts occur, and there is relationship or attitude to the particular thought. We can be aware only of our momentary experience. We are never aware of anything other than ourselves. The paradox of awareness is that we think we are aware of a world outside of ourselves. Awareness is us noticing ourselves. We cannot be aware of objects, events, or people, only of our relationship to them. When we see, we are aware only of our own seeing. When we hear, we are aware only of our own hearing. Our senses sense only our senses. We never *know* anything outside of ourselves. Our assumptions about a material world separate from ourselves are pure illusions, the material of dreams.

Awareness of relationship between people and things is awareness of the interconnectedness of the events that take place in our own nervous systems. We are creatures of our own experience, since we do not know anything outside of that experience.

Coming to the understanding that we are awareness becoming aware of itself is the development of wisdom. Acceptance in equanimity of this paradox allows us to live sanely. Struggle against the awesome knowledge that there is nothing but our own experience is the beginning of disease. Therefore, the only real cure for our illness is the practice of becoming aware of ourselves.

Awareness is the key element in the maintenance of personal health and the healing of illness. Awareness is an active knowing. It is neither a thought nor a feeling about reality, but it is the appreciation of all the combined thoughts and sensations comprising the experience of being a human life form.

Human life is a succession of thoughts and sensations that arise and pass away. Thoughts occur in the context of the mind. Sensations occur in the context of the body. However, the mind and the body cannot be separated. They exist together simultaneously in time and space, not as fixed, separate events but as the continually changing, somatic form of human life.

Human awareness happens as an experience in the context of time and space whereby attention is given simultaneously to thought (concept) and sensation (feeling and emotion). When this occurs, there is a deep understanding of the unity of the human form with its surrounding environment. This understanding can be, in itself, healing.

◎ FORM AS PROCESS

We human beings, especially those of us who live in Western society, tend to recognize, at any given time, only one aspect of our experience of being human. We fragment our lives in this way. Some people identify themselves with thoughts and tend to think that they are their thinking. Others relate more to physical sensations and tend to identify themselves as bodies. The truth of our existence as somatic form is a greater whole than these artificially separated parts. The mind and the body should not be separated in our understanding because they are not separate in actuality. This fragmentation of identity is a lack of awareness, and such a lack is the condition in which dysfunction and disease occur.

The greater whole is not a static, solitary event. Rather, our somatic form is a process and an ongoing movement comprised of two interrelated and simultaneous aspects that we call mind and body. The motion of the mind aspect is a continual arising, coming into existence, and passing away of thoughts, remembrances, and fantasies that we call thinking. In the same way, the body form is a continuous arising and passing away of all sensation, whether it be seeing, hearing, tasting, smelling, touching, or the constant streaming and rumbling of the body's bio-electric field, which is our emotional reality. The fact that these movements occur simultaneously and relatedly in space and time allows us to perceive them simultaneously as the unified somatic whole that we also call the mind-body process. Awareness is this perception of the whole somatic form and is the source of our sense of vitality and well-being. It is also the origin of our deepest religious feeling and sense of awe over the mystery of creation.

◎ CONTRACTION AND EXPANSION

Life is movement. We experience a continuing, alternating rhythm of contraction and expansion in our whole being at all times. At any given time in normal functioning, we are experiencing one or both of these two movements. Our cells expand and contract. In the work of sensing environment and producing appropriate motion, muscles expand and contract. The brain expands and contracts within its covering membranes. Spinal fluid does the same, and the heart is the prime example of this basic pattern of alternating movement.

Psychologically, we experience contraction of our state of mind in times of anxiety and depression. Anxiety is a contraction reaction to the changing situations around and inside of us. The feeling of well-being is associated with movement toward expansion, as is the full expression of our emotions. When we feel good, we "open" to the world. We speak of our heart being "open" when we feel love. We say our heart is "closed" when there is the absence of good feeling. Movement is the change between expansion and contraction, and it occurs as change in the direction of closing or as change in the direction of opening.

Stagnation in either a state of contraction or expansion, without the natural movement to the other state, eventually results in illness. A continual state of resistance to the alternations of expansion and contraction, in both mind and body, will eventually manifest as deterioration of body tissue and impaired functioning of the whole somatic human form. Resistance to life movement creates tension and disease in both body and mind. A cramped muscle is an extreme example of contraction. A tension headache is the end product of chronically contracted neck muscles. An atonic, expanded colon, unable to contract, cannot discharge waste and disrupts the normal physiology of the body.

In our world, movement is always accompanied by inertia or resistance to movement. This occurrence of movement and resistance together is a natural law in the world of form. When excessive resistance to movement occurs in the physical aspect of our somatic form, we see stasis of function and atrophy of tissues. In the mental aspect of our somatic form, resistance to movement is characterized by a clinging, grasping quality of the mind. There is a tendency of the mind to resist the expanding and contracting pulse of life by clinging to emotional attitudes, particular people or things, to beliefs, to "pet" ideas, to any desire, or even to a favorite physical sensation. This clinging quality of mind is the basis of all attachment to neurotic defense mechanisms and, in its extreme, produces what we call mental illness.

For instance, if one experiences a devastating loss of a loved person and there is willingness to experience the contractions of grief and anger fully, and then to allow the "letting-go" of that person, completion of the grief occurs, and there is release of attachment. When there is, in contrast, resistance to the entire experience and grief is not allowed expression, the attachment to the lost loved one is not loosened. Grief is followed by apathy and depression. The entire life experience then is one of stagnation in contraction. We say the person is depressed. Actually, there is resistance. Restoration to health (release from depression) would occur with acknowledgement and expression of grief. Expression is the restoration of movement.

◎ CONTRACTION AS ILLNESS

Usually, the resistance to movement that we observe to be the source of illness arises simultaneously in the mental and physical aspects of the somatic form. In other words, one does not cause the other, but dysfunction happens in the whole form. Most commonly, the lack of movement occurs as a fixation in the contracted state. For example, a middle-aged and successful businesswoman came for treatment of severe and debilitating low back pain with limitation of movement. Her success in business was the result of her emotional and mental attachment to achievement and her obsession with control of herself and those around her to attain power and material success. Her pre-occupation with these ideas can be considered a contraction of her mental form and an imbalance in her mind/body process. The imbalance was a chronic condition caused by her continual involvement with thought images at the expense of attention to her body.

She was not aware of the severe tension in her lower spine until she experienced severe pain while lifting a suitcase in a busy airport and was unable to straighten her back or to walk. Upon examination, it was found that the ligaments, tendons, and muscles surrounding the lumbar spine were in a state of extreme contraction. The bending and lifting movement had been too much in such a rigid system, and something "had to give." Ligaments were torn and bleeding, and vertebrae were moved just slightly out of optimum position for smooth functioning. Movement in her lower spine had stopped in a contracted state and, as a result, had impaired efficiency of movement in her entire body. The method of healing would have to be effective in converting stagnation into movement. Her mental and physical contraction, common symptoms in this society, would have to be released into expansion in order to restore function. This kind of holistic intervention must act on the entire somatic form in both its physical and mental aspects.

◎ AWARENESS AS PRIMARY HEALING AND THE VALUE OF BARE-ATTENTION

Before discussing the intrinsic healing power of awareness, we should describe in more detail what awareness is and how it happens. As we said earlier, awareness occurs when attention is given simultaneously to thought and sensation. This idea of simultaneity is important, since attention to just thought or sensation alone is not awareness in and of itself. (Although, as we shall describe later, it is the focusing of attention that is the method of producing awareness.)

When true awareness happens, there is a momentary dissolution of excessive resistance to movement and change. With this dissolution, opinionated ideas and beliefs about oneself are dissolved, as are the attachments to particular sensations and emotions that accompany such beliefs. Also dissolved is the "holding" in of muscle and connective tissue that coexists with constricting ideas. Understanding of the true nature of self, of the personal relationship to people and the environment, arises. This deep knowledge, in its profundity, is healing. Awareness heals.

The essential ingredient for the development of awareness is the ability to pay *bare-attention* to the natural unfolding of life's phenomena. It is also the *method* of gaining awareness. Bare-attention is the observation of our experience without attempting to control what happens with our opinions, preferences, conditioned or prejudiced ideas, or analysis of the experience being observed. Bare-attention is just what it says: attention stripped of any extra covering. When practicing bare-attention, we can observe the energetic pulsings of our inner life, visceral movements, tissues contracting and expanding, and thoughts coming and going. With time, we can recognize recurrent patterns of sensation and thought that are characteristic of our individual experience.

The practice of paying bare-attention is not as easy as it sounds, however. We humans have a strong attraction to a kind of walking sleep state where the effort of paying bare-attention is replaced by ignorance of what is going on around and within us. Our minds are incredibly adept at diverting our attention from its focus. We have desires, fatigue, irritation, or any number of distractions to divert us from paying a simple attention to what is happening. Much of the time we do not want to know our internal state. We are afraid of the *intensity* of thoughts and sensations, and we turn our attention willingly or unconsciously away from them. It is then that the conditions in which illness flourishes can continue without obstruction.

In order to learn the practice of bare-attention, concentrated focus is necessary. The object of focus may be either thoughts or the stream of sensations that are continuously occurring as mind/body process. Directing attention to a particular sensation or to a particular thought or repetition of thought is the method of developing concentration. Concentration of focus on thought or sensation leads to the perception of both as they occur simultaneously in our experience. Perception of both is awareness.

The value of concentration of attention in regard to awareness is that concentration results in a calming of the random activity of the discursive mind. When the mind's usual ceaseless and diverting chatter has subsided, even slightly, there is an increased ability to attend with clarity. As the mind's frenetic activity is quieted through effective concentration, the body tissues relax also. With relaxation of body and mind, the information about our biological life that continuously comes to consciousness is obvious. The act of concentration is, therefore, healing in that it enhances interest in life and the capacity to fully experience ourselves. A good teacher or healer knows the healing power of concentrating the attention and will teach a client how to develop and use it.

Awareness is a uniquely individual experience. Each of us has our own understanding and our individual perceptions. Our senses, which can be the mediators of awareness, bring information to the central nervous system. This information can be the focus of attention. The way in which this process happens is the same for all of us; however, the content of the information we receive is individual.

The process of becoming aware is on-going and never-ending, but if we postulate a beginning, it occurs when we perceive that something is happening. A particular physical sensation is a good object on which to focus attention. For instance, a light touch on the skin stimulates a sensory organ. This stimulation is actually a kind of disturbance. The excitation or disturbance is mediated as energetic change to the receptor cells of the central nervous system by way of the sensory nerves. This traveling of energetic impulse occurs through a system of enzymatic and neurological steps that is awesome in its precision and specificity. Each minute step is crucial in itself and dependent on the step that precedes it. The occurrence is sometimes likened to the flow of impulse through electrical wiring. Once the stimulation originated by touch has traveled through the peripheral nerves of the body and is received by the central nervous system, the physical stimulation has become information and has potential to be an object of attention in the form of sensation. Then we can say, I am experiencing sensation. Sensation is happening now. The information received is further delineated in the brain so that we can know the sensation to be of a particular quality and occurring in the left arm rather than in the leg. The sensation, if it is to be consciously noted before passing away, must then become a dominant (foreground) event within the field of our attention at the moment. When we direct attention to our senses, we are developing interest in information that is continuously emerging through the modality of that sense.

Awareness as Healing

In the case of the businesswoman whose low back injury we described earlier, the method of intervention entailed the necessity of restoring mind/body harmony. Since she was already preoccupied with her mental life at the expense of body functioning, our method of healing began with directing attention to her physical state. The painful injury, with the intensity of sensation involved, had already started this process in a natural way. Knowing that concentration produces relaxation of body and mind, making awareness possible, we chose to use the intense sensations of contracted and injured tissue as the beginning focus of attention.

By using light touch, we began to coax her reluctant attention to the injured area so that relaxation might begin. To do this, we had to encourage her to perceive the discomfort as intensity of feeling. When beginning relaxation occurred, we further sharpened the concentration by using deep touch to exaggerate and call attention to the pressure sensations of the deeper contracted tissues. In this way, we began to introduce her to the value of bare-attention with body experience as focus. In addition to light and deep touch, the same concentration method was practiced using slow, active and passive movements, stretching postures, focused breathing, and later spinal manipulation to restore vertebral alignment, all designed to coax attention to the body's contracted areas. Through these methods, she began to recognize contraction as tension and tension as resistance to movement.

Deep touch in the muscles of the lumbar area, performed gently and to the limits of tolerance, produced prominent sensations. These sensations became useful repeatedly as focus for instruction in the use of bare-attention. The relaxation and "letting go" of tension aroused her interest in the phenomenon of the change from contraction to expansion. The sense of well-being that accompanied the change supported her interest in this process of healing.

She became vitally interested in the health and well-being of her whole somatic form and began noticing with increasing skill the effect of her mental attitudes and her emotions on her physical experience. She also noticed her tendency to deny the importance of the biological life of her body. She saw her need to control, her orientation toward achievement, and her unwillingness to experience fear, sadness, and anger. When the tissues relaxed in the healing process, the emotions released were powerful and cleansing. Her whole body relaxed in relief from the chronic tension. Intense moments of awareness, and profound understandings of herself as mind/body process, reinforced her growing interest in restoring balance in her life.

The treatment worked. It was not all accomplished in one consultation visit, but relief from the severe contractions began immediately. The course of healing and relaxation occurred over a four-week period, with weekly visits and specific stretching and movement exercises practiced daily between visits. A simple diet of raw salad greens, steamed vegetables, and juices augmented the treatment plan. Although the healing process demanded enormous effort on the part of the client, the lasting effects on her whole lifestyle made the treatment preventive as well as curative, a benefit that cannot be gained by the use of symptom-suppressing drugs.

The difficult part of treatment by these natural methods is that the newly developing awareness focuses on what is immediately present as sensation, and the experience most evident in the beginning is the unpleasantness of pain. The immediate task is to show the client that pain is not an experience to be avoided but rather one deserving of attention.

SECONDARY HEALING ASPECTS OF AWARENESS: RIGHT ACTION

At times, our ability to utilize the primary healing nature of awareness as a self-help tool is exceeded by the seriousness of the situation. Sometimes the symptoms of discomfort are already so severe upon recognition that we do not know what to do. At this time, the secondary healing aspect of awareness becomes important. Awareness can lead to right action. Seeking expert help from a healer is right action when the situation appears to require more information than we presently have.

A film director, intensely occupied with his work, failed to pay attention to the first signs of his illness: small amounts of dark red blood appearing in his stool on several occasions. Perhaps his preoccupation with his artistic projects distracted him from taking immediate action on the painless bleeding. Several weeks later, he experienced wrenching lower abdominal pain, and the severity of the pain could not go unnoticed. Realizing that the situation was beyond his means to cope with, he consulted a holistic healer, who directed him for further internal diagnosis. The medical doctor recommended immediate surgery, which was a difficult and complicated removal of part of the descending colon. The small amount of bleeding had announced the presence of a large, cancerous growth. Right action in this situation led to radical intervention and to the man's good health, now, seven years following the surgery.

Observation of physical symptoms is not the only event that may lead to right action. Observation of emotional pain and dissatisfaction in the quality of life are indications of imbalance, also. Simply noticing frequent thoughts and feelings of dissatisfaction will not necessarily result in primary healing. The noticing of dissatisfaction or discomfort is sufficient, however, to move us to search for more information and more instruction, if we are willing to take action. Attention to physical symptoms of pain or the body's improper functioning, and attention to dissatisfaction with our attitudes toward life (even in the absence of actual illness), make right action possible. A well-trained holistic healer can respond with valuable guidance in either situation, but the observation of the need for help is the first step toward seeking it.

For example, a salesman came for consultation. He was a large, robust, intelligent man. According to usual medical standards, he was in generally good health. But he had complaints of feeling alienated, lonely, and repeatedly unable to establish fulfilling and intimate relationships with other people. He experienced little joy and noticed his growing apathy. He was depressed and discouraged and came to the consultation with the intent of improving the quality of his life. Although he complained of vague pains in his upper chest and neck, there was no clearcut symptom of physical disorder requiring intervention at that level. His sense of humor and ability to describe his existential situation were intact; however, he lacked a passionate presence in his manner and in the quality of his contact.

His body, particularly the upper torso, was heavily armored: his musculature hard and inflexible and the superficial tissues tense. The expansion of his barrel-shaped chest was limited even with deep breathing. The musculature of his abdomen was taut and hard. The movement in his hips and pelvis was rigid so that he walked with short and ungraceful steps. His thighs were hard, and his legs were thin and underdeveloped compared to his upper torso. His feet were pale and cold. He lacked spontaneity in his facial expression, and his eyes were wide, staring, and deeply set, with an expression of worry and sadness. Even so, he was an ordinary, functioning man, successful in his business and the father of several children. To the unpracticed eye, he would appear strong and healthy.

We noticed that he had a subtle, characteristic way of breathing, and frequently he seemed to "reach" for a deep breath as though he could not get enough air. This grasping for breath was accompanied by a slight twisting, rocking movement of his head and neck to the left. He said he had noticed this habit of breath movement for a number of years. We decided to investigate this peculiar movement further, since his complaints of vague pain were associated with his neck and upper chest. The focus on this movement as a method of investigation was a way of working with the obvious. When viewed through the practitioners' bare-attention, the movement was seen as a prominent symptom of his discomfort.

Our intent was to enhance his awareness by using a method of conscious exaggeration and repetition. Exaggeration is a way of making the movement or action more obvious. When an action or movement is performed with repetitious regularity, and the process observed with bare-attention, the movement or action takes its place as an expression of the entire somatic form. It assumes meaning in our awareness in much the same way that repetitious chanting, mantra, or prayer heightens awareness in a spiritual practice. This investigation was carried out in a quiet, supportive environment with the client reclining on a comfortable body-work table. The contact between the client and the practitioners engendered trust and acceptance, without which investigative work of this nature would not have been possible.

We asked the client to perform the exaggerated head and neck movement with his breathing in a repetitive pattern. After doing this movement for a while, he said that he was aware of a feeling that he could not get enough air. He experienced fear, a hunger for more air, and a feeling of suffocation in his chest. By this time, he was deeply involved in the therapeutic experience. We asked him to continue the movement, and he appeared to enter a kind of reverie. When asked about his experience, he said, "It's like I am about five years old. I remember lying alone in my bed often, rolling my head back and forth and singing to myself, 'Wowie, Mommy Daddy.' I think I was afraid and overwhelmed by loneliness. It gets foggy."

Then we asked him to roll his head back and forth and sing the childhood chant, "Wowie, Mommy Daddy." He was embarrassed. With encouragement, and after several false starts, he began the movement and chanting. Very quickly, there came a great welling-up of emotion: sobbing, choking, and intense feelings of grief. These were followed spontaneously by great outbursts of rage, hitting the table with his fists. Again, he dissolved into sobs, which subsided into soft crying and deep, full breaths. This melting of resistance resulted in a softening and relaxation of the musculature of his upper chest and neck.

When asked about the experience, he said that he had remembered his loneliness and isolation as a child. His father was a violent man who often beat him during his bursts of anger. He spent his childhood in terror of provoking these outbursts. Lack of loving contact with his mother deprived him of protection and support. His brothers were as terrorized as he, so the children were left to comfort each other as best they could. During this work, he had re-experienced these strong emotions which he had not allowed full expression of as a child because of the contractions of fear. He had defended himself against these emotions with the rigid armoring of his whole body.

This cathartic breakthrough marked the beginning of new depth in his therapy. The awareness experience opened up new attitudes toward his life. He understood that his anger and grief were associated partially with his childhood fears of his father and lack of contact with his mother. They were problematical in his present life by the way they influenced his relationships with people now, preventing open contact and the giving and receiving of loving attention. The more he was able to accept, non-judgementally, his biological emotional life, the more able he was to interact with compassion.

We should emphasize that this kind of dramatic catharsis, described in this man's case, is not the end-point of intervention but rather marks a beginning to the learning of new attitudes. This learning is the work of continuing investigation of the therapeutic relationship between client and practitioner. Further work develops awareness of the interrelatedness between the body experience and the mental/emotional life. This is the gaining of self-knowledge through the practice of awareness.

◎ CONCLUSION

The two people whose illnesses and treatments we have described presented themselves with widely differing complaints. And yet, the method of therapeutic intervention in each situation was essentially the same and depended upon a systematic awareness practice. In both situations, the method used involved touch and movement for directing bare-attention, in a concentrated way, directly into the area of discomfort. In both cases, the therapy was holistic in that the methods involved were concerned equally with the mental and physical aspects of the client's being. They were treated as a whole, somatic form; as a whole person.

With the development of concentration, relaxation of the body's tissues occurred. Relaxation of the mind's attachment to certain emotions and attitudes occurred, also. Movement was restored in both body and mind. Healing followed. The body has the innate ability to heal itself under the proper conditions, and relaxation is one of the conditions. Nutritious diet and positive mental attitudes are also conditions for healing. In both of the cases described, the process of developing awareness was accompanied by a lively arousal of interest in the experience of the clients' own biological and somatic existence. New attitudes of appreciation and compassion for themselves and others were important aspects of the healing process. Also, for both clients, the holistic approach to their illnesses was effective because their disorder had not progressed to a point where tissues were permanently damaged. The practice of awareness must be an accepted part of daily living so that the inevitable imbalances in our lives can be restored to harmony. Right action can prevent irreversible damage, and right action can be only a product of awareness.

Unfortunately, many of us learn awareness solely through the experience of an illness. It is as though the wandering attention is finally forced to focus on our immediate experience by the nagging pressure of discomfort. Resistance to concentration on actual experience can result in a lifestyle based upon the idea of illness as a recurring theme. We all know people who seem to be endlessly obsessed with sickness and repeated visits to many different healers. Each visit seems to feed the preoccupation rather than alleviate concern. The healing session becomes another step in perpetuating the style of living based on illness.

Hypochondriasis (preoccupation with one's own physical health or lack of it) is essentially an *avoidance* of body/mind awareness. The concentration involved in moment-to-moment attention is either too much effort or would bring unwelcome knowledge of the suffering itself. Many people want to escape their suffering without experiencing it first.

The struggle for awareness and the resistance to it occur simultaneously. We want the healing that awareness and open contact bring, but we do not want to experience the disease. One is not possible without the other. "Being saved" from illness without having direct knowledge of the illness occurs mostly in the imagination. Maybe the imagination is strong enough to heal, but usually it is not. People become healed when they are able to experience the disease and then truly desire to be free of it because it is unsatisfying. Illness occurs in our lives whether we are aware or unaware. But if there is awareness, we are better able to deal with the illness.

8

THE ENERGY DIMENSION

AL BAUMAN

There are no healers! In ways sometimes strange and often mundane, we humans help each other by pointing to doors—exits from our prisons. Those who walk through the doors are called "healed," and those who don't are in a state of dis-ease. The dynamic is that of friendship, an interesting combination of tenderness with cannonballs of truth—truth being my point of view as opposed to yours. Involvement in life has to do with energy and movement. Life is inconceivable without energy and without motion; to stop either aspect means sickness. My exploration is in dimensions of energy and movement: depth, extension, the movement of emotions, qualities of energy, how energy manifests, how colors change in nature, and so on.

Energy manifests in radio, television, electric lights, sex, and emotional responses. Energy can be considered as something more than a working word. It is a real thing. "Energy" is a current world concern in terms of supply and demand for running machinery, in terms of the care and continuity of the planet, and in terms of the dangers of atomic explosions and other atomic emissions. It is also a concern in personal experiences of lack of energy or of explosive releases of energy through violent expressions and through revelation, and in considerations about longevity and death.

The manifestation of energy is in the rings of trees, the spiral shapes of cone shells, the movement of clouds, and the communication of expressive intent through combinations of sounds. I know of my energy through my experiences of being tired or lively and through the sensation of energy streaming within my body. As a child, I spoke of tiredness that streamed out of my feet at night. Later, energy made itself felt in many dimensions in my body, sometimes as warmth and glowing, sometimes as uncontrolled twitching after a very exciting or suspenseful or dangerous event. The arts, too, can be experienced as energy in movement and pulsation. Dance is energy moving in space; music is energy manifest as sound; and painting is the movement of color in space.

Perhaps the sun sends energy to the earth rather than light. The higher up we go in space, the darker it gets. The energy of the sun meets the energy that surrounds the earth, and the dawn breaks—explodes—every morning. Illumination happens when the energy of the sun meets the energy of the earth. When illumination occurs, its by-product is heat. In the body, the atmospheric energy is ingested from the sun's rays and through food and chemical processes. Then, the energy manifests in heat and temperature differences and actual illumination of the field of the person.

Healthy, energetic functioning in a person implies unimpeded energy flow throughout the body and the ability to use energy as needed in work and in emotional expression. Motility is having the power of spontaneous motion, the ability to react spontaneously. Reactions express the energy generated for an action. When a person is healthy, the energetic aura surrounding his or her body is full, about four or five inches or sometimes larger, and one can see a wave-like movement of the energy. That general movement is in a kidneybean shape around the person's profile: up the back, over the head, down the torso, in at the naval and down, in a longitudinal axis. The person experiences energy in a flow called *streaming* and, fortunately, can nowadays mention the streaming more freely without being called schizophrenic and being put away. The streamings are experienced pleasurably; there is a feeling of unity, and the body moves as a whole. Also, in health, people respond very quickly with emotions: anger is available to them as protection; they can reach out easily; they are tender; and their expression is lively and spontaneous.

In loving, beginning sensually and extending to sexually, there is a build-up of energy, a feeling of intensity. The streaming becomes stronger. There is a sense of being taken by the streaming to the point that we can't sit by and observe. It becomes so intense at the climactic point that a person feels a moment of unconsciousness. A sensation of warmth spreads over the whole body, and frequently after the orgasm, involuntary twitchings appear in various parts of the body— shoulders, face, legs, belly—almost like horses twitch their skin when a fly lands on them. This twitching is not very different from the way the belly moves in crying or laughing. The release of loving occurs when the energy fields of two people meet, like the illumination that occurs when the energy of the sun meets the energy of the earth: an explosion.

My nephew was born in the New York Hospital, and it was a long and difficult birth. I saw him when he was six or seven hours old in the nursery. He was put in front of a glass window. When I walked up to the window to look at him, he began twitching madly. So I stepped back and, when I was as far back as three feet, he stopped twitching. If I went closer again, he started twitching again. There was some quality of presence (which can be seen as an energy phenomenon). As my field approached his, he began moving uncontrollably.

Trembling reflects energy passing through the musculature as, when putting an electric charge through a frog's leg, the whole leg twitches. When vibration goes through the muscle easily, then the vibration is like a streaming of heat. When there is great resistance and the muscles are very tight, then the twitching becomes very large and sometimes painful. It is the energy attacking or breaking through where the musculature holds. This holding of the musculature can be felt by an outside hand; the muscles gather almost into clumps and sometimes coagulate to the size of a walnut. When energy hits these, the vibrating can be rather violent, like a tantrum with pounding and large movements, or the movements may be subtle. Sometimes this movement is accompanied by a specific story that includes an event, sometimes not. One of the ways that I look on such uncontrolled movement is that those expressions that have been inhibited have been remembered by the systems of the person and by the muscles. So the unconscious may be the memory that is held in the organs or the muscles of the body. After release, motility is increased. The ability of the body to respond spontaneously – in the muscles, the emotions, and the organs – is heightened. The twitching loosens the muscles, and there is a general sense of well-being.

My experiences with energy and its manifestations were clarified and explained by Wilhelm Reich, and his theories and discoveries are the take-off point for my descriptions of energy in holistic medicine. Reich called the atmospheric energy "orgone" and postulated that organic matter attracted and *held* energy, while inorganic matter attracted and *repelled* energy. Therefore, by layering organic and inorganic matter, an accumulation of energy could be effected. He built accumulator boxes on this principle and found that there were temperature differences between layered and unlayered boxes, indicating through the measurement of heat that an energy differential also existed. The accumulator principle is the single best treatment of burns that I and my physician friends have encountered. For burns that happen in any kitchen, the immediate application of a layering—for example, an iron pan covered with a cloth—over the burned area often cures the burn within 15 to 30 minutes. The burn breaks the envelope that contains energy. The application of an accumulating device functions in the same manner as a blister but speeds up the process.

The most dramatic experience I have had with burns was when I fell against a steam pipe, after showering in my New York apartment, and scalded my back in a diagonal line from shoulder to buttock. I immediately sat in a large accumulator box, and within half an hour, the burn was healed. The skin remained tender during the evening hours when I went to a party, but I was able to move about and dance with ease.

◎ THE ENERGY FIELD

I see the energy field of the body first as a flow similar to what we see when looking at the profile of a mountain or on the horizon when looking over the ocean. This flow has been called the "aura" and shows itself more or less intensely, with brighter or duller lumination, close to the body or extending out four to five inches or more. Sometimes it has color—mainly light blue, red, yellow, and green. Sometimes it is interrupted by black streaks.

Ted was a man of about 50 years. He had been a downhill ski racer, and, though he gave up competition many years before, he was still trim and athletic. He played table tennis at a semi-professional level, ran three or four miles daily, and was an active competitor in paddle tennis. He was an educator with an extensive number of publications and original work in developing tutorial communities within public school systems to his credit. Ted had lived with ileitis for 20 years, so he was especially careful of diet.

One evening toward the end of a group session in which Ted had expressed much rage, a red aura—a sharp line running vertically along the lower left side of his body—caught my eye. The sight persisted, and, though Ted appeared at ease, I heeded my vision. I put my left hand on the red line and held my right hand in his right hand, as in a handshake. My aim was to draw energy from the red area and to place it in his arm where he could move more easily than in the lower torso. In about four or five minutes, Ted complained of strong pains in his right shoulder. I did not tell him what I was doing, so there was no suggestion involved. The red line was now gone from the field and the ileitis was gone after that day. He no longer lived on bland foods; he ate and drank in moderation, finding discomfort only when he ate particularly spicy foods and when he had been inexpressive in stress situations. Both conditions were easily self-remedial.

There are some simple ways of measuring auras. If you put some graph paper up on a wall with simple backlighting, and you stand a person in front of it, you will see almost immediately how the light is very bright at the edges of the person. The outline is not sharply defined, but it is a bright light which changes in size. The outline can be traced on the graph paper in the dimensions of the aura. It will be clear where the illumination is broken—either a sharp line or a space will be seen. The discontinuity indicates a place of blocked energy. The effect is not simply from the light hitting an inanimate object because it differs from person to person.

Claudia was a pianist preparing to appear with one of the major symphony orchestras. A young professional well on her way to a full career, she persistently faltered in one passage of a Mozart concerto. I was working as a music teacher and coach and saw no indications of musical problems. My observation of the energy field around her head showed a full field except for a sharp break—a black streak extending out from her chin. The break in the field indicated to me a tightness in the chin and possibly the jaw. The quality was of "holding on." I rubbed her chin vigorously until the black streak disappeared. With that, the specific performance problem disappeared. Dissolving the holding on with her chin revealed an attitude of praying, a philosophical and spiritual problem. Further steps in our work together fulfilled and expressed the attitude of prayer and released playing blocks.

The degree of personal presence is another indicator of energy. Everybody presents themselves, but the qualities of presence are very different from person to person. If a person comes on only as aggressive and straightforward, something seems a little cockeyed. There is perhaps an element of sadness or shyness that the aggressiveness is covering. For the charismatic, strong person, the energy field is almost always enormous, sometimes extending as far as a foot or two feet out from the body. In people whose presence is slight, the energy field is frequently so contracted that it is below the skin. The person does not feel touching or, instead, feels pain.

Eleanor, age 35, came to me as a referral from her psychoanalyst. She was blocked in affect, unable to express anger and, therefore, showing her emotions in distorted, exaggerated expressions. Eleanor had never been allowed to sleep alone as a child. Her mother or grandmother slept with her until she was 16. It was like they sucked her dry; she never developed a sense of her own independence. She resented it and contracted. Her body showed almost no energy field, and it was impossible to touch her anywhere, not even as a simple gesture, such as putting a hand lightly on her shoulder as a greeting, without causing her pain. The energy field acts as a buffer, both protecting the skin and introducing it to outside elements. Eleanor's orientation was "suspicion," waiting for attack yet unable to respond to attack. To bring her energy field to the surface, I worked with her body at a distance of three to four inches away from the skin. Work consisted of moving my hands around the body contours as well as shaking my hands to vibrate the field toward and away from her skin, a gesture similar to bouncing a ball very quickly. There were many cold areas. One can differentiate heat emissions from the body by approaching the skin slowly with one's palms, much as one would carefully approach a metal that was anticipated to be hot. At one point, prematurely, Eleanor tried receiving a gentle, pleasuring massage. Far from pleasure, she experienced the massage as agonizing pain with fantasies of murdering the masseuse. It took 10 sessions of vibrating the energy field before Eleanor could accept being touched. The process of unarmoring and reschooling followed.

The energy field translates the stimuli that come to us into emotions and into sensations of being connected with life, whether those sensations are violent, fast, slow, strong, or tender. The energy field, then, is the medium through which the stimulus comes and is translated into the sensory organs of the body. When that field is not present, people are suspicious and paranoid. People with no fields are always suspicious because they know they feel pain, but they don't know where it comes from. These people tend to have very darting eyes. The field is like the antenna of bugs. It is especially protective of newborn children.

Mark was a concert pianist, an acquaintance who was becoming a friend. I attended a concert of his and saw an alarming energy phenomenon. As he played, the field around his head was intensely white, giving a circular halo effect to the whole head. Suddenly, there was an explosion of light emanating from the top of his head. The explosion lasted a few seconds, and then the field diminished considerably. I was worried and went backstage after the concert to congratulate a very tired musician. The energy event stayed with me. I slept poorly and called early the next morning to Mark's home. He had been taken to the hospital with a ruptured brain tumor. He did not survive the operation.

CHANGING THE FLOW OF ENERGY

In my work with people, the first thing I look for is a general liveliness, a sense of vitality. I note particular expressions, both on the face and in the body. These expressions range from total contraction or resignation to exploding rage and many steps in between. I see a general demeanor first. Then I glance intently, yet casually, over the body, without concentrating on any space or place, and hope the body will show itself to me. It soon becomes clear where the main expression is focused. Some people are very focused in the eyes, others in the belly, and so on.

When I find the place where expression seems to be focused, I look at the person's general field and usually find a counterbalance for that spot. If there is a very intense energy in the eyes, for example, then there may be another such spot in the thighs, the belly, or somewhere else, that is also intense. There seems to be a pairing of energy spots, as if the head reflects parts of the body. Following this, I assess the flow of energy. I sense hot and cold areas of the person. By looking or by running my hand around about four inches above the body, I can tell where there is more heat emanating and where less, where there is more and less energy.

With some people, as my hand comes near the body, involuntary movements begin. When I hold my hand just four inches above my client Kitty, for example, her whole chin starts to shake. Her eyes are closed, and she doesn't know I'm there. Her chin is an area where the expression is very intense, but held, without expression. Muscles start to twitch, and sometimes her joints move. In another client, when I come close to her chest, her legs start moving. In some people, when the two energy fields of my hand and their body meet, something physical happens. These are people whose energy fields are very alive, so I can work directly with that field and frequently never touch the body.

We can consider energy by using the symbol of a stream. We can dam it up, or we can increase the flow by adding more water to the stream or by digging out part of the downstream bed so that it drops more quickly. We can increase the flow or change the flow by various modifications. Likewise, we can change the flow of energy streams in the body. People can learn to do this voluntarily by drawing energy from parts of the body. For example, if the chest is high and stuck, and the breathing is difficult, we can take energy away from the diaphragm. Then, as the chest drops, the energy flow moves down. I do this by using my hands, and anyone can do it by bathing, using water.

When energy moves easily, breathing is easy. I learned, when I met Reich, that there is no such thing as dysfunction without an interruption of the breathing pattern or an inability to breathe however we need to. We can work both ways, from energy to breath or breath to energy, and approach either one from the other.

Erich, a 43-year-old psychiatrist, was born in Vienna and left when it was threatened by Nazi invasion. As a small boy, he was sent off to another country, later to be met by his parents. In the course of our work together, one constant in Erich's facial expression was tics around his eyes. Whatever was released and whatever expressions became part of his spontaneous being, the eye tics remained. At one of our sessions, I increased the energy potential around his eyes by vibrating the energy field with my hands and by having Erich breathe with a regular pumping action and maintain the charge without expression. I fully expected that the release that would result from the excessive energy buildup would be tears. To my amazement, Erich burst into laughter that was full, infectious, wild, and free.

He recalled an associated story. Ten years or more before this session, Erich's father had died, and Erich, of course, attended the funeral. In the intensity of the situation, he had an acute awareness of the ridiculousness of much of the ceremony around the burial. He was also charged with pent-up emotions about his father's death. He suddenly burst into laughter. Ashamed that he would show this, he covered his face with his hands. Surprised, he heard people praising him: "How moved Erich is; he is rocked with tears and crying over his father's death." People had mistaken the muffled sounds of laughter for crying. This was the origin of the tic. The conflict that showed in his face through the involuntary movements around his eyes and in his cheeks had to do with laughing or crying. Crying and tears were acceptable and approved; laughter was not. Add to this experience the family background of escaping Hitler with many wounds to show, the heavy weight of re-living the escape, and the relationship to the holocaust, and the lesson was clear: cry, don't laugh. The release from this bondage gave Erich an infectious, spontaneous laugh that he had not experienced since early childhood.

At one time, my awareness of the whole was through movement. I was a professional musician, and I wanted to know what makes music move. As a child, I whirled in circles as in ballet turns and then gave these whirls content by dancing my impressions of people in motion. One early dance was about New York traffic cops, who seemed to have to face in four directions at once. Another dance series had to do with the movement of baseball players and combining the moves of all the positions on the baseball field.

Later, I realized that if someone has an area of intense energy, the movement in that area is likely to be different. For example, a guitarist came to me several years ago for treatment. He had 19 years on the police force in New York, was about to retire, and wanted to continue as a musician. The difficulty was that he held the guitar very tightly because he held it like a machine gun. He could play well enough but could only play for three or four minutes until his arms and chest tightened. He had spent 18 years on the rescue squad taking people out of water, getting cats out of trees—a benign policeman. Someone caught on to this fact and reassigned him to two years doing some of the dirty work: going out in a prowl car, being out in the streets, and so on. When we saw what the problem was, I asked him to show me how he behaved in a patrol car, and we walked around the room. Nothing moved but his eyes. He didn't want to see danger; he didn't want to see anything. If he did see something, he jerked around to his partner and told him to drive the other way. This is not uncommon. Policemen don't want to get killed. He was holding onto his guitar—or his machine gun—for dear life. We worked with the movement through dancing until his arms released; then he could play the guitar.

What makes a dance move? Another person who came to me was a dancer from Martha Graham's group. She had just come from a world tour. She danced in pain, and she said, "You know something about movement that I don't know and Martha doesn't know." With this dancer, every step was a new dance. She didn't understand the movement of emotions—that an emotion or a movement leads to another movement. The question we worked through was not what the movements are but how the connections are made. Like the movement of a good angry fight leading to tenderness, if it isn't a good, full fight, it leads to spite. There are progressions of emotional states and movement states.

Vibrations, too, can excite movement within the body. The vibration of a sound we create can hit the body of another person and can be experienced as pleasant or unpleasant. I recall a period of teaching music at an Eastern university when I played a recording of Varese's "Ionization" for a class. The students were so shocked by the sounds that they fell into raucous laughter, and some fell out of their seats. When I asked if the music had reached them, they all agreed that it had *not*. It had only knocked them out of their seats! Music that violated their traditions shocked students into knowing and dealing with their own sensations.

It is also possible, and very useful in dealing with energy phenomena within our own bodies, to find our own sounds. The sounds for each person are different. I have experienced certain vibrations in the organs of my body that I know are in tune to D minor. The voice is a primary form of being in the world. Just as vibrations can release the musculature any place in the body, so these vibrations create a sound.

Caroline was three months old when she was brought to me. Her parents commented that she was a perpetual whiner, at three months a well-accomplished complainer. The child's skin reflected her energy field. The skin was mottled and splotchy, with patches of red and a general criss-cross pattern of red and white. The energy field was intense. The heat emanating from her body could be felt at a distance of five to seven inches, but the field was discontinuous, running hot-cold, hot-cold. Though there was a general liveliness about the infant, her chest was held unusually high for someone so young. I helped depress the chest in exhalation, and I encouraged longer exhalations. The rhythm of breathing stabilized at a ratio of about 1:4, inhalation to exhalation. Caroline began to whine and complain immediately, but after a few moments in the new breathing pattern, she burst into furious rage. The mottled skin became a smooth pink and the energy field took on a soft, warm glow, without great intensity, and a lovely, light blue color with no visible interruptions.

This infant had not been allowed to wait for anything. No sooner had the well-intentioned parents heard a beginning complaint than they would pick her up and satisfy whatever need she seemed to have. At home, she never experienced her full expression of demand. Within a few minutes after the new breathing pattern was established, Caroline was fast asleep. I then asked the parents to have a session, but they were reluctant with the child in the same room. "The noise will be frightening, she will awaken." They had lived in an aseptic, sound-inhibited environment for three months! We proceeded with a session in which there was much noise and loud yelling. Caroline opened her eyes once, looked around, smiled beatifically, and went back to sleep.

Two general streams create sound in the body. One stream comes from over the top of the head. Then as we breathe, and as the chest or the whole front collapses, a certain amount of energy comes out. There are eddies, almost a spiral movement. This stream meets the second stream at about the upper lip. The sound that comes from over the head excites the whole area around the eyes and the sinuses. It is the sound of crying, while the sound that comes up from the chest is the sound of roaring. Great singers have both streams combined, like a double helix of energy. Certain singers have more of one than the other; for example, Jan Pierce, the opera singer, is a wailer with a crying voice. There is no strain on the throat at all, so those with the crying voice can sing forever. Then there are singers who primarily bellow, and they don't last terribly long. It is a marvelous, rich sound, but it is not modified by the upper stream. When the two streams come together—Barbra Streisand in popular music is an example— then the voice is useful in any dimension.

A symptom arising from impeded energy flow along the longitudinal axis of the body and the consequent bursting out of dammed energy through the skin is eczema. Dennis, in his late twenties, exhibited large areas of rashes. Dennis' redness and scaliness showed on his back in a triangular pattern from a line across the shoulders to a point midway down the spine. His eczema had been present for nearly 12 years. Dennis' symptoms were advanced and startling. Though his back was red and hot, he felt no heat, and the energy field was very shallow. He was an inexpressive person in general demeanor, with the expressionless character of his face covered by a full beard. His body was of a sallow complexion, and he had a variety of disorders ranging from hypoglycemia to kidney dysfunction. The combination of heat and limited field told me of an expression of spite—a poor, revengeful substitution for anger and rage. His back was so scabby that it was impossible to touch it directly. I massaged the energy field, instead, at a distance of about two to four inches from the skin level. As his expressions of anger erupted, they led almost at once to an attitude of inhibited reaching. At the expression of both of these emotions, the rash disappeared in about four weeks. New skin has grown over the old wounds.

Cathy was a 32-year-old asthmatic with hay fever and numerous assorted respiratory allergies. I observed intense red coloring around her neck with a brightness and depth that seemed to express embarrassment. Strangely, the field around this area was very weak. Her skin showed large, red blotches going up to the chin, around the back of the head, and part way down into the chest. I know that emotions and inhibitions related to respiratory disturbances are expressions of longing and the interruptions of these expressions. I remembered Janet, who had come to a workshop with bronchitis accompanied by an uncontrollable hacking cough. I had asked her to put herself into a physical posture of reaching—arms extended, head rolled back, chest depressed—while baying like a dog to the moon. In Janet's case, the coughing had stopped immediately, and the pain of inhaling had subsided over the next three hours.

With Cathy, the situation seemed more severe. Since asthmatic wheezing, like stuttering, can be completely bypassed by singing, I asked Cathy to hum and then to sing. This excited the field around her neck. The intense redness moved deeper into the chest area. The expression on her face now looked like her lips and chin were reaching for a kiss. Humorously, but seriously, I suggested that she do a lot of kissing accompanied by extending her arms to express the yearning that started in her chest and moved up to the chin and mouth. She practiced in the session and returned a month later with no symptoms of asthma and no hay fever reaction to the pollen of that spring season. In fact, she boasted that she could approach plants and bushes and inhale the pollen without reaction. There was a slight return of the allergies in the next month, and the intense redness around her neck continued. It seemed to abate only when she sang, and the thought struck me that her asthma had something to do with not being heard. We went into long, loud, extended song—or what passed for song. The asthmatic attacks have not recurred, though she does worry about possible recurrence. The specific expression here involved power and self-assertion. As she expressed "Hold me," her usual body sweatiness and the paleness of her lower torso disappeared.

The observer is part of the energy phenomenon. So, the observer must be able to describe himself or herself. While I am working with a person, I know how I am feeling, what I am going through, and what my general state of well being is. As I work with a person, I will feel some things that are strange to me; for example, I may suddenly get a pain in the left side of my head. I know that's not my pain because I never hurt there. When I suddenly have a pain or a burst of warmth, then I know the person I am working with is doing the same. I go to that spot in the person and work to get any problem moving. Probably 99 percent of the time, this approach is accurate. This is not magical. It is the illumination that occurs when two energy fields meet.

I see blocking of energy as a universal problem that can go in one of two ways. It can appear as a feeling of needing to explode or kick the dog—the five o'clock disease in every American family, the time when the mother is yelling at the kids, and father comes home and tries to yell at everybody. The blocking occurs because energy input has not been expressed. Because some people freeze energy rather than express it, the other way of blocking is to go into depression, for depression is frozen emotion. A common way of trying to get out of the frozenness is to shoot up drugs, drink alcohol, or leave.

Stuckness is not having too much energy; rather, it is not accepting the natural flow of energy. One has been highly stimulated but then fails to move with the energy. We should feel moved, feel a streaming sensation. For example, when we go to a concert, our manners say, "Don't jump up and start dancing in the aisles." So we wear our best clothes and behave properly, but what we really want to do is jump up and down, yell "Bravo!" and go up on the stage and shake everybody's hand because the music is exciting. But we don't express it. Instead, we try to verbalize it, which only gets rid of about five percent of the energy. Treatment, therefore, involves accepting the flow of energy, allowing movement and excitement.

Anyone can do the kinds of treatments I have talked about for himself or herself. The person can get in touch with energy flow and be aware of energy movement. The person can use nearly any health discipline to approach energy. With a headache, for example, we can learn where energy gets stuck. The streaming over the head may stop at the cheekbones and upper lip. As the energy hits that blocked place, it bounces back, like water hitting a seawall. One of the best ways to cure a headache is to give someone else a massage. Almost always, this moves energy out through the arms. Bathing can also move energy. People can consider nutrition from the point of view of energy, recognizing food as an energy source and regulating food intake in terms of feelings of energy within.

Another simple way of changing energy flow in the body is to soak the feet in epsom salts. Energy moves down quickly because water is a powerful grounding force. Energy always moves from the smaller field to the greater field. If a person stays in a hot tub or with his or her feet in hot water for only a short time, the energy balance is changed. The energy streaming in the body moves more fully down the front. If the water doesn't draw too much, the flow downwards is increased, and the person can feel very good. But if a person stays too long in the hot water, then he or she loses energy.

Another way to change energy is to gain energy through motion, as in exercise. The best way I know to gain energy in motion is through pleasure. We usually learn pain and the disciplines of pain very easily. Then we build up defenses, hold our breath, and so on, to avoid pain. The greatest disease in this society is pleasure anxiety, so one of the largest industries is entertainment, a substitute for pleasure. As our genuine pleasure becomes more profound, we feel happier with it, we move energy more easily with pleasure, and we feel excitement, warmth, and contact. We're healthier.

9

THE SPIRITUAL DIMENSION

AYSE WHITNEY

The word *spiritual* is mysterious to the multitudes—mysterious because most of us have explored it very little. In learning to understand our spiritual dimension, we are really becoming conscious. To become conscious is to become aware of our inner self and our vital connection with the world around us. In the effort to become conscious, we make the mystery of spirituality less mysterious to ourselves. The terms *psychic healer* and *spiritual teacher* also have an aura of mystery; they imply one who tells a fortune that an ordinary person cannot know or one who sees light that the ordinary person cannot see. But psychic healers and spiritual teachers do nothing more, in healing people, than make them conscious.

When we begin to pay attention to our inner world at the deeper levels, we are beginning our training in the spiritual dimension. We train to make ourselves conscious of exactly who we are; we are even conscious, ultimately, of the belief system in which we function and of the fact that we have created the system. The training slowly teaches us to balance our feelings and intellect. We learn to understand, then, the nature of thought form; we are not overwhelmed by our psychic experiences and abilities, and we know their purpose.

The human soul is a realm of thought forms animated by feelings. In this realm, what we think becomes our palpable reality, externalized around us. There is not a standard psychic realm. We each have our very own heavens and hells that we create by the way we think. Our objective reality is the momentary manifestations of our way of being mentally. More precisely, our mental way of being is animated or enlivened by our desires, by our feelings. The soul is not just the mind or just the emotions: it is an interaction between the two. Without consciousness or awareness, we notice happenings in the mind rather than in the soul. The mind must be enlivened by the charge of feelings for there to be an experience of soul or psyche.

The spiritual dimension is reached by a redirecting of attention. The mind thinks constantly, in a linear fashion; it is full of its thinking. Entering the psychic realm takes a very slight tilt of attention. The mind stops being preoccupied with its "busyness," changes focus, and reflects the subtler realm. When we stop thinking constantly and are still, when we allow ourselves to *be* and our mind to reflect this "way of being," we take our first step in learning about our soul.

Psychic phenomena, also, can be understood as a shift in attention. For example, a woman recently had an out-of-the-body experience, and her reaction was, "Amazing! What is this?" Later, she sat with a young man who told her that he was leaving his body. He was very frightened because he couldn't find his way back to his body.

Like the woman, he was creating a problem out of none. Being out of the body is nothing but a change of focus. All that had happened is that both people had concentrated away from their bodies.

Nothing is invented. Newton did not "create" the law of gravity—the apple fell and gravity existed before Newton. He "saw" gravity. So it is with the psychic reality. We are psychic whether we think we are or not, but we cannot experience the psychic realm until we bring our attention to it. Once we admit into awareness the psychic reality, as a dimension of our whole being, that reality becomes active in us. Most of us have attended to our outside life, but our psychic life is unknown. Understanding the psychic life is a bit like going into a jungle, so we need a clearly-defined structure, like a map, to explore its territory. The structure may take the form of a philosophical or religious belief system, or it may be a daily practice like meditation, yoga, or chanting.

Through, for example, disciplined meditation, we reach an experience of our mind, of our consciousness, which is quite different from a concept or an idea about the mind. This experience brings with it an intrinsic, organic knowing, which again is different from an intellectual knowledge. And the organic knowing brings to us an experience of being spiritually rooted, an experience of knowing we are a vital part of the universe.

People who spend time in meditation eventually become conscious of psychic abilities, like clairvoyance, clairaudience, precognition, and other kinds of extrasensory perception, rather naturally. These abilities exist for everyone in some capacity as part of the spiritual dimension. The development and use of psychic abilities really depend on the past patterning and experiences of our soul, in its emotional component and its mental conceptualizations. The specific qualities and content of the experience can vary immensely from person to person. One person may be extremely intuitive or precognitive, while another is clairaudient only. So, there are many ways that each of these psychic capacities occurs.

In general, clairvoyance is being able to see into the world within oneself. It is not the same as seeing forms in the outside world, using eyes. Clairvoyance requires surrender, in the sense of becoming a part of the world within, so the inner world is real. Seeing begins with a kind of "feeling tone." Then a vision of sorts arises. What is actually seen—the form, shape, color—will be different for each person.

Clairaudience is hearing in a similar way, but likewise, it is not the same as hearing an outside sound. It is like a vibration that happens throughout the body and forms words in the mind, similar to words being heard. An example of the way this happens is that one may experience auditory vibrations that shape into something like a voice, which conveys a message. There may be sounds other than voices for another person.

Precognition is being able to sense a fact that might or might not emerge into objective reality. It is sensing the presence of an event that could take place. The existence of these facts or events is already present and obvious to certain parts of our psyche, but we must be able to surrender to the depth of our feeling to sense them. So precognition is opening ourselves to realities that do exist under or beyond objective reality.

Any of these kinds of psychic experiences or capacities usually conveys a message or a sense of our direction and place in life. The message comes from within ourselves. All of these capacities involve a relaxation of the mind and a turning of the awareness to a subtler realm, the world underneath the conceptual. It is allowing a wash of another reality to emerge yet never negating the objective reality. To receive inspiration from our spiritual rootedness in the universe, like a plant receives sap from its roots to feed the flower, is the highest spirituality. This experience leads to the organic knowing of our spiritual roots. It is precious in that it allows genuine inspiration in the soul of the human being.

If we do have some kind of psychic ability, like clairvoyance or precognition, it does not necessarily follow that we are rooted or spiritual. In fact, to be spiritually rooted and inspired, we need not have these other psychic abilities.

Spirituality is not acquired by wishing to have psychic powers. These powers come as side effects as we struggle to live in accordance with the inner teachings, the lessons we receive from exploring our inner selves. The development of psychic powers by themselves can, in fact, be dangerous; these capacities can be misused like a scalpel in the hands of somebody who is not a surgeon. The danger with developing psychic powers separately, without an encompassing spiritual practice, is that these abilities are then perceived through the mind instead of through the soul. They are practiced without the underlying purpose of inner growth. We soon get into the narrow world of psychic powers without spiritual sensitivity. In going to a psychic to seek special powers, we digress further from growth into a creative, loving, independent entity. The psychic abilities are sideline capacities that may or may not emerge during exploration and training of the soul. They are not of major importance in the spiritual dimension as a whole and should not be the center of focus.

A BELIEF SYSTEM AND STRUCTURE

Our consciousness functions through a structure. What we think of as real is real for us. We are creators of systems of belief, of our own versions of reality. We need these belief systems to provide a structure to enable us to function in the everyday world and in the inner world. For people who experience the psyche but do not have a belief system that has a use and interpretation for this reality, the experiences seem very dispersed and dreamlike. At some point in our growth, the Buddhists say, we strip ourselves of all belief systems and unite with the big sea of consciousness, the realm of universal knowingness. In the meantime, popped out of that big sea like an individual droplet, we need a belief system to structure our reality.

The belief system provides a structure within which to explore. We need not strip ourselves of belief systems; we do need to learn the nature of the mind and the nature of reality. To function consciously, we need a system. Belief systems are both a way of describing and a way of creating form out of the essence of life. In developing a belief system, we create something out of no-thing, really. From the ground of consciousness, feelings flow into form, and then concepts encapsulate forms.

Belief systems are useful and necessary, but no one system is absolute. In order to use belief systems with a healthy attitude, we have to learn to respect other people's systems, to accept alternate realities within ourselves, and to build bridges between those realities. Accepting a belief system or building a structure takes time and flexibility, and at points along the way, it can be confusing.

When we start to explore the psyche, it is at first tempting to project onto the spiritual realm the same hardness and rigidity we find in the material realm. This is an unhealthy approach to the psychic world or to psychic healing, and we can end up creating a rigid belief system. In the psychic realm, we truly are what we think. We can get stuck on one viewpoint for a long time until we find out that, the more we think in a certain way, the more it is going to be that way. There is nothing to prove us wrong. We seek the evidence to prove ourselves right, and the evidence comes.

Because it is only when a question is asked that the person has started wondering, an ancient axiom for teachers who help us explore the psyche is not to answer unless asked. If someone is thinking in a certain way, especially in psychic matters, he or she will prove the teacher wrong every time if the teacher talks at the person. Every system has its logic, and the person moving within the logic of his or her system proves himself or herself right.

This is why guidance and a reliable meditation practice, as part of our structure and belief system, are necessary as we develop our spiritual awareness. Without them, we just add to our troubles by creating misconceptions. With the practice, we put to good use the new material we experience. Gradually, we become more creative, flexible, open, and responsible in our thinking and in our way of being.

The development of character is also important in our spiritual practice. We must understand and control our feelings in our relationships with others, and we must control the visions that are the expressions of feelings when we develop inner sight. We cannot allow ourselves to be inundated by these experiences or visions. Lack of control can extend to psychopathology, as with people who can hear voices but cannot stop the voices, and people who have visions but cannot stop the visions.

In esoteric practices, we can create a form, even a negative form, without letting it overwhelm us, and then disintegrate it. This form may be an image or an obsessive figure that somehow haunts us. As we integrate the negative energy of this image into ourselves, accept it as part of our own shadow, the vision completely disintegrates. If we do not know how to handle our feelings and do not also have a system that explains these occurrences, we can be overwhelmed. These things are as real in the psychic dimension as an object in the hand is real. With a practice that includes daily discipline, working attentively on the mastery of emotions, all that we see in the inner realms are thought forms charged with feelings.

As the soul becomes real to us, and as we become aware of its rules and how it functions, we are naturally motivated towards right ways of being. We begin living in a way that is right for us. We stop living in a personal hell and start living in our own heaven. This experience begins to define a path we are choosing to take.

The way to the inner realms, called the *path*, must be followed in a controlled, structured way because what we want to develop is a positive psyche, a healthy soul. Just as there is a fine line between the genius and the lunatic, there is also a fine line between a person with a positive, strong psychic channel and somebody who is completely overwhelmed by the events of the inner world. If we do not have a structure, an inner discipline, we will be flooded by the sea of the unconscious.

◎ THE PATH

The path is like the belief system in that we create it. We have to re-member that the belief system is created out of no-thing *and* that it is extremely important. Similarly, in a way, there is no path. The path lies where we are right now. We find ourselves asking questions like, "Why am I on earth?" "Where have I come from?" "Where am I go-ing?" These questions the mother and the father cannot answer any more, or society cannot answer any more, or if society does answer, we do not buy the answer. We start feeling lonely. We pretend we're okay, but we are not, and slowly, the pressure of this loneliness introverts us. Through loneliness, we face ourselves one to one.

We can also get onto the path by a big catastrophe in our lives. Wars often start people on the path because questions arise: "Why on earth are we having a war? What is it worth?" The catastrophe can just as well be very personal, as in the loss of a loved one, or a period of psychological depression. From this loneliness, we become intro-verted enough to sense the validity of our question and the yearning for an answer. We come to the point where we feel that if this answer isn't there, life is not worth living. Out of our yearning, we create an ideal. "I have these questions, and they are very important for me. I need this answer, this 'God,' this certain type of feeling. If there be not *this*, then nothing has meaning." This yearning creates a "magnet" in ourselves that draws and unifies a lot of our psychic energy. At that moment in our lives, synchronistically, we start meeting persons, sit-uations, events, or books that teach us.

We start being carried along, and we are tested. Many books, paths, teachers come our way, and we are tested in our discrimina-tion. The yearning, the inner quest, carries us until, finally, we hit upon something that resonates clearly with us. Whatever this is does not have rationale. A guru doesn't have to come in yellow robes. Our grandmother, a friend, a book or a technique can start us practicing. We live in remembrance of that sense of resonance or connection. We keep it in the forefront of our minds. It becomes a touchstone for our give and take with life. Whenever we have ups and downs, this qual-ity or sense starts directing our emotions. If we have a technique, like chanting, meditation, or bodywork, we practice the technique.

After a certain point on the path, we need a personal teacher who, for a while in our lives, can truly share his or her practice with us. This person may not be a world-renowned guru or teacher, but it is usually someone whose form is a channel for the essence that we have sought. The person resonates with the essence that we have yearned for and perhaps named "God." Such a relationship can carry us through a lot of personal work in a short time. Yet, while we are in training with our personal teacher, we are also preparing ourselves for the time we have to leave our teacher, to retain the essence in our own hearts.

CHANGES IN HEALTH

Once we have begun the path, certain kinds of change take place as we move from confusion in our lives to more clarity. Initially, the chaos may become greater. For the first time in our lives, we are studying our own minds and learning the way we think. We soon become aware of how rigid our concepts are. We believe we have certain possibilities and impossibilities in our lives, and we live according to these possibilities and impossibilities. Some of these conclusions make us constricted in our behavior, and some create emotional turmoil within us. We can even feel how our bodies become tense from the emotions. Between the dawning awareness and the eventual change that we have to undergo, we enter a period of purification.

There is a cleansing process that we must go through, which may be different for each person. Some of us become more sick than we have ever been before. In the short term, there may not be an amelioration. There may even be a healing crisis—seen as an illness. In the long term, when the soul is made whole, the body feels better, too. Sometimes we will find that a part of our psyche will cause great problems, and this may not change for years. But at a certain moment when, through our practice of mindfulness, our character has become strong enough to carry the challenge and the temptations, an opening will occur. A whole Pandora's box opens. If we have not pushed it, and it has opened naturally, we will have the strength to transform its contents.

We may think our practice is bad because we are not getting physically healthy. But, as long as we do our best to live mindfully and have love in our hearts, our growth will continue. We get better, but in God's time. The changes that happen quickly are the easy ones. We do get a bit more relaxed, more independent, but the real trouble spots change slowly.

The biggest changes come when we are not so anxious about ourselves any more. We understand that our problems will go on. If we want to expand our consciousness, we have to deal with fear, despair, chaos, and ignorance; and we understand that it is no big deal. We integrate and balance "It is no big deal" and "It is very important." We feel but are not overwhelmed by the feeling. We are beyond being overwhelmed, and our perspective has changed. It is on this attitude that all further exploration of inner realms is based. We become normal, natural persons. And, soon after this change, we start to serve humanity.

◎ THE HEALING

In the beginning of the counseling session, the spiritual healer is not as concerned with the person as with being very open, without any preconceptions as to what will happen. The healer must check any kind of movement such as a wish to fix the person or to succeed in the counseling. What the healer brings to the counseling is his or her own practice in openness. It is in this openness that the healer finds love. Although the term *love* might not be used, to be open without preconceptions is an act of courage that can extend only so far as the capacity for love exists within us. It is the courage of love that enables us not to cringe in fear or in revulsion but to stay in relationship, which is, of course, the experience of love. Thus, when the healer sits with a person, he or she brings to the situation as much of a relationship as is possible without any ideas that would split the counselor from the person or the situation.

The crucial link between the counselor and the person is the healer's capacity to feel and be open to parts of the person that he or she cannot relate to as yet because those parts are too tight or too hard. The person is less loving or less open towards certain parts of his or her consciousness and tends to be unaware of these parts. The healer, though, is open to them. In this relaxed atmosphere, the counselor feels certain events without getting stuck on them and brings about a release of emotional and spiritual blockages in the person. The counselor can release these concerns to become not as tight or important as the person deems them. On another level, through openness, the healer sees movement where the client cannot, possibilities where the person sees impossibilities. Out of this kind of insight, the healer communicates with the person verbally, usually through questions dealing with the *persona* first, and feeds the person his or her own answers back from a different angle.

The counselor's openness also creates in the person a trust, a relaxation, and a feeling of being accepted that allows the person to touch the places in consciousness that otherwise he or she might be too lonely or too scared to touch. In a true sharing of the meditative experience, the healer touches areas confronted in his or her own practice. This experience is described both by the Buddhists and the

Christians in the person of the bodhisattva, who stops and exists on the earth level until all sentient beings are liberated, and of the Christian, who stops for his or her brother-man or sister-woman. These figures have a magic in them that heals the soul. Without techniques to fix us, they heal just by being there with us and for us.

The magic is that the counselor is simply present at a level that the person is as yet afraid to touch. The healer goes beneath the person's consciousness into what the person feels as a hell and touches the person there. The counselor reveals it to the person as less than hell, and the healer loves the person there. The person feels the healer's very knowingness and presence revealing something about that area of the consciousness that the person didn't know could be true. The counselor relates to the person at that level. Then the person is not afraid, feels possibilities, and sees the dignity within. Once the person can be touched at this level, the organism takes over and the healer doesn't need to fix anything.

True spiritual or psychic healing is most clearly summed up by the statement, "Put love in your heart, stretch out your hand, and heal." This kind of love doesn't come by taking psychic development courses. It comes only by truly receiving our daily bread in the form of our karma and dealing with it from the viewpoint of dharma (the teachings of life). The certain attitude toward the daily bread or life circumstances turns obstacles into stepping stones and creates in our psyche and our circumstances an openness that leads to enlightenment.

An hour of psychic counseling can range from an outwardly mundane give and take, to the healer sharing certain intuitive and clairvoyant perceptions of the person's state of health and circumstances. The healer usually does not go to a session ready to receive these impressions but rather goes completely open for whatever is to happen. A tremendous number of phenomena can take place without the healer searching for something specific.

Certain things do occur repeatedly. One of these is that, through a certain way of looking at people, the state of the health of the person's subtle body becomes apparent. It is perceived not as "out there color or shape" but as a kind of "feel-see" or "think-see." This is an organic kind of knowing that uses the counselor's whole organism, not just the eyes. It is a bit like having an X-ray diagnostician in the counselor's organism when he or she "sees" into the astral, the subtler energy, body of the person. The psychic counselor can see the stress areas, areas that are overworked, and can usually see disease or blockages occurring before there are any physiological changes. Thus, he or she can deal with the disease at the more fluid, subtle energy-body levels before damaging physiological changes occur in the more concrete material of the physical body.

The work that the counselor is doing, apart from its intrinsic healing nature, is diagnostic. The counselor can usually determine what kind of occurrences or processes in the person's psyche are causing these diseased, blocked areas. When these are mentioned, the person will say, "Aha, yeah. I do feel that." At a certain level in himself or herself, the person is aware that something is happening in an area. The counselor can then give intuitive psychological advice or nutritional advice and suggest vitamin supplements or the appropriate kinds of bodywork. The counselor can advise the person to go to other practitioners of preventive medicine or to see a chiropractor, masseuse, acupuncturist, nutritionist, or medical doctor.

Part of the counselor's work is to find the most suitable means of health care for people's personalities. Some people are willing to start meditating, but others are neither ready nor capable of doing so. For these people, it is much better to start on the more physical levels, so the counselor can suggest gentle massage, acupuncture treatments, or nutritional change. Even for those ready to take responsibility for spiritual changes, physiological ramifications make help on the physical level necessary, at least at first.

HEALING AT THE BODY LEVEL

An example of bodywork used in spiritual development is called *Yoga of Light*. It is derived from Hatha Yoga and developed by this author into its present form. Yoga of Light is a simple approach. It fills the mind with the feelings from the body. When, without concepts, we listen to the feeling tones from our body, we cannot escape the realization of our emotional or spiritual pain. An ever-deepening awareness of this pain also reveals to us what we do to bring the pain about. We do not conceptualize anything in this practice; we just remain aware. When awareness deepens enough, change occurs because we see clearly that we must change to be rid of the pain and its cause. Sometimes, this deepening of the awareness can take a tremendously long time and can be tested by mental arguments. Or the pain and the awareness may be so great that they quickly cut through any mental arguments, and we make very rapid progress towards a happier, more rooted way of living that is compatible with who we really are.

The work is done with the help of the breath and a "reflective" awareness. We very gently find where our breath is and let ourselves be completely guided by the movement of our breath. This not only calms the mind but also opens a door to the experience of the body. The mind "reflects," without labels or judgments, the feeling tones arising in our embodiment.

The body contains all the mystery that we need to open up to; all that we need to relate to in reaching enlightenment. There is no separation between the mind and the body; they are made of the same basic substance—consciousness. In the West, we have strong minds and, being intellectuals, we tend to objectify even our own bodies and alienate ourselves from our surroundings. This leads to an atrophy of the "sensing" abilities. We like to think we cannot or should not be affected by our circumstances, that we must be able to survive in negative surroundings that could be too loud, too crowded, or destructive to our well-being. To survive in such surroundings, we have to close up, to repress the input. We dampen our senses. When we are cut off from our senses, we are not fully conscious or aware. With this kind of bodywork, the person has a practice that will allow him or her to expand the consciousness.

Yoga of Light also heals the body-mind split through development of compassion. The very act of being with ourselves is an act of friendship. As we start realizing that we can't fix ourselves, but we can *be* with ourselves lovingly, then the act of being with ourselves, our embodiment, gets gradually more refined. As this practice becomes more refined, it opens the heart. We can never be with anything or anyone completely if our heart center is not open in compassion. Even in meditation, we can go into our heads, especially in the beginning of the path, and create a further split from our body. When we are trying to be very good, we can mistake who we would like to be for who we are. Who we are is locked in the body, and as long as we do not tune into our embodiment, we will not develop openness and compassion. Bodywork reminds us who we are; we cannot run away. We are with exactly who we are, not daydreaming but in the present. Learning to accept our various states, we gain compassion for ourselves. Seeing our pain in others, we find compassion for them.

In the beginning, the bodywork gives more pain than pleasure. The movements are done gently—they have to be done gently—and the directions always include the words *kindness* and *gentleness*. People are encouraged to get in touch with their breathing and to develop a non-competitive attitude. The pain arises when people attempt to be gentle and then find how competitive they are, how cruel they are, how unfeeling they are towards their needs and their being. It is an interesting sight to see people "married" to a movement that reflects to them exactly who they are.

Movements express inner experience. We can open ourselves to these experiences through awareness. We take one movement and gently do it, or hold it in a fixed way for several minutes, and then slowly get out of it. We then sit with the sensation, the reactions that continue happening within our consciousness. In this kind of work, there is absolutely no good or bad. From boredom to bliss, the movement is designed to create reactions within us. Our work is to be present with ever-keen awareness while experiencing whatever state of consciousness we are in at any moment. Breathing, chanting, and visualization exercises, together with sitting and walking meditation, expand and complement the movement.

Yoga of Light exemplifies a spiritual practice that heals the body-mind split and develops compassion, which makes the person down to earth and does not take him or her away from life. It helps the person lead a more sane, practical life and be more fully in life. The person slowly thaws out what he or she finds are frozen areas. With teachings given in such a practical form as bodywork, spiritual work becomes practical and approachable.

◎CONCLUSION

We cannot force our attention to turn towards our soul. Usually, what first motivates us is pain. A continuing awareness of our psyche teaches us the nature of the pain, how we create pain for ourselves, and how we can heal the pain. At a certain point, our awareness leads us to experiencing the natural fact of our being, and we understand that we are rooted in the cosmos, in the world soul. We can be inspired and fed emotionally, mentally, and physically by these roots. When we find inspiration, we change from the motivation of pain to the motivation of knowledge of happiness. Thus changed, our practice continues. The psyche is not tangible; it is not solid. We make the psyche. May we make it healthy and happy. May we make it well.

10

THE EMOTIONAL DIMENSION

JOHN S. SMOLOWE, M.D.

Seeking enlightenment, a traveler sets out to climb a certain renowned, remote mountain. Although the way is long and arduous, he perseveres, for he has heard that, if he climbs long enough, he will reach his goal. Suddenly, moving downhill out of the mist, a second man appears, accompanied by three large, black dogs. So strongly do they strain against their leashes that the man almost runs to keep up. It appears that he walks them, but perhaps they lead him.

The two travelers stop and exchange details of their routes and their aspirations. The second man is not returning from an uphill journey; he is following a downward path to fulfillment. The dogs that lead him darkly on the run are the emotions.[1]

In holistic theory, emotions are valuable, even such "negative" moods as anger, fear, and guilt. In holistic healing, the practitioner avoids the authoritarian stance and gives few orders. The client takes responsibility. Instead of prescriptions, the client receives guidance to an inner sense that can discriminate healthy food, exercise, breath, etc., from unhealthy.

EMOTION AS AN ORIENTING, HOMEOSTATIC FACULTY

Emotions and moods* are crucial tools of this discrimination. Take our stance: we lean forward eagerly, back off cautiously, and jump joyously. So we name with moods our orientations to the environment.

Holistic theory also emphasizes the ability of the organism to heal itself. The tendency to return to equilibrium after a disturbance is termed "homeostasis." Our emotions are often homeostatic. After the death of a loved one, for example, we withdraw, cry, and get angry. This grieving process, built in through millions of years of evolution, discharges the pain and restores equilibrium. When challenged, we can grow angry automatically. Assertive and powerful, we move forward to dispel the threat. Certain moods feel distasteful for good reason: they arise as we discriminate which foods, exercises, and relationships do not fit our needs.

Take nausea, for instance. Though infants regurgitate spontaneously, with no apparent discomfort, most adults experience nau-

---

*The two terms sometimes differ in meaning. "Mood" connotes a state; "emotion" an event. Moods tend to last longer. For a discussion of function, mechanisms, and components, as in this chapter, the two terms are interchangeable. "Feelings" include not only moods and emotions but also sensations and intuitions about other people or situations, for example, "I have a feeling that they're going to get married."

sea and vomiting as unpleasant or embarrassing. Physically, vomiting is certainly homeostatic: the organism rids itself of something taken in that does not belong, and nausea warns us to prepare to vomit. Further, nausea signals us that we have taken in either too much food or the wrong kind of food.

Nausea also functions as we take in concepts. When sports columnist Lowell Cohn cannot swallow a certain opinion, he becomes nauseated.

> I found myself agreeing with him, 'Oh yeah, (the coach) is so nice,' I said to myself. And then I was almost overcome by a feeling of physical revulsion, the feeling you get when you know you're lying to yourself.[2]

Jean Paul Sartre, in his novel *Nausea*, describes the pervasive state of nausea that can arise when an individual works too long at a job.

> Mercier was going to Bengal on an archaeological mission. I always wanted to go to Bengal and he pressed me to go with him. . . . I was paralyzed, I couldn't say a word. I was staring at a little Khmer statuette on a green carpet next to a telephone. I seemed to be full of lymph or warm milk. . . .
>
> And then, suddenly, I woke from a six-year slumber. The statuette seemed to me unpleasant and stupid and I felt terribly, deeply bored. I couldn't understand why I was in Indochina. . . . My passion was dead. For years it had rolled over and submerged me; now I felt empty. But that wasn't the worst: before me, posed with a sort of indolence, was a voluminous, insipid idea . . . it sickened me so much I couldn't look at it. . . .
>
> I pulled myself together . . . and answered dryly: 'Thank you, but I believe I've traveled enough, I must go back to France now.' Two days later I took the boat for Marseille.[3]

Nausea can emerge when we join a group in which we don't fit or when we stay too long in a relationship or activity that once felt right. Nausea then warns us to leave.

Guilt, too, can be homeostatic. We all have values, direction, and goals. The ability to know which actions feel ethical is healthy. To act ethically, we must be able to recognize when we have made mistakes, when we have gone against our values. Much guilt, it is true, is destructive self-criticism, but often, guilt is the recognition that we have violated our own ethics. Then, guilt is a re-orientation, teaching us how to act ethically the next time.

◎ EMOTION AS A MULTIDIMENSIONAL EXPERIENCE

Emotion can be experienced directly. We can know that we are angry without first checking for angry thoughts. But emotion is not a separate, detached experience; it colors the other dimensions of the person.

In the *abidhamma* or Buddhist psychology, the mind (the knowing faculty) is clear. Various types of mental factors, such as greed and attachment or concentration and mindfulness or the emotions, color the mind. For a time, all sights, sounds, and thoughts are known in that color.[4, 5] In the West, Heidegger[6] explicates mood as *befindlischkeit*, the sense of ourselves in a situation. A holistic concept, it refers not just to an internal feeling nor just to a perception of the outer world but rather to both, " . . . without or before dividing them."[7] Consider, for instance, the colloquial use of "Where are you?" to mean "How do you feel?" Or consider the answers "I feel far away," "I feel lost," or "I feel on top of the world." "Understanding," writes Heidegger, "is always moody."[8] "Understanding is never free-floating, rather always *befindlisches*."[9]

So mood manifests in many personal dimensions. In sadness, for example, the corners of the mouth turn down, the eyes tear, the shoulders slump—the whole body takes on a heavy downward directionality. We feel "down." At times like these, even our vision changes. Things seem somber, gray, and dull. The world looks blue.

> The pockets of the great coat and pockets of the trousers . . . are blue like the empty sacks they resemble. There is a hint of blue in the toothbrush glass. The loneliness of clothes draped over the backs of chairs is blue; undies, empty lobbies, rumpled spreads are blue, especially when chenille and if orange; not body warmth or body smell . . . no—blue belongs to the past—to the minutes after masturbation, to thought, to detachment and removal, fading, to the inside side of sex and the self that in the midst of pitch and toss has slipped away like a lucky penny fallen from a dresser.[10]

When we are sad, songs telling stories of sadness or loss come to mind. Memories of old, sad times, times that carried the same emotional tone, come back as visual images. Digestion slows down. We walk more slowly and talk more slowly. We withdraw from new activity and turn towards other people for comfort. And we are aware of the sadness. "How am I? Glad you asked; yes, well, yesterday I was kinda gray, but today I'm downright blue."[11]

In anger, the body spontaneously feels more energetic and surges into movement. The muscles tense as if practicing action. If the facial expression is not masked, the lips snarl, the eyes glare, and the jaw thrusts forward.[12] The eyebrows lower and knit together, while the eyes open wide to glare or narrow in a piercing stare. Vision becomes vigilant—more selective and focused rather than open and accepting. Imagery of striking and hitting arises unsought. The heart pounds, and the breath deepens. The fists clench. Thoughts arise: "I'll kill the SOB!" Intentionality is clear and focused on meeting the threat, on planning action. And we know we are angry.

This diverse, yet coherent, way that mood manifests itself supports a multidimensional view of a person. Body structure, movement, breathing, energy, senses, imagery, intentionality, emotion, spirituality, the capacity for relationship, self-regulation of diet, awareness—each of these is a facet or aspect of the whole person. Further, each is a faculty; a resource or capacity. We can experience such faculties directly (unlike a construct such as "superego"). These faculties function simultaneously and collaboratively in health. They all malfunction in illness.

When we observe any one dimension, we find that the other equally important dimensions are linked to it. Further, as we highlight one faculty and make it foreground, the others recede. They seem like components of the dimension we are studying. When we dance, energy and affect seem like aspects of the movement. Here, as we investigate emotion, imagery and posture will seem like components of the moods. Our perspective is important. When we are looking at the whole person, emotion becomes one of many linked dimensions. When we are looking at emotion, the other dimensions become components of mood.

◎ EMOTIONAL DYSFUNCTION

Emotions do not always function adaptively. Indeed, the term, "emotional problems" is often used synonymously with "psychological problems." Adaptive emotional expression can be altered in several ways. First, a person can voluntarily inhibit an emotion. Some people are restrained in confronting challenges; for example, they might inhibit the spontaneous arousal of aggression. If they are habitually timid, they end up living in circumscribed safety, as in hen-pecked submission to a spouse.

Other people are detached. They may notice the components of their emotions but they do not notice the whole or the orienting homeostatic function. They do not "belly-ache" about a problem; they take Tums. Meursault, in Camus' *The Stranger*, is alienated from his emotions:

> I explained that it had no importance really, but, if it would give her pleasure, we could get married right away. I pointed out that, anyhow, the suggestion came from her; as for me, I'd merely said, 'Yes.'[13]

He has moods, but he recognizes them either not at all,

> Through the wall there came to me a little wheezing sound, and I guessed that he was weeping. For some reason, I don't know what, I began thinking of Mother.[14]

or else aesthetically, as if he were watching a movie rather than acting and responding,

> It was an effort waking up that Sunday morning . . . My head was aching slightly and my first cigarette had a bitter taste. Marie told me I looked like a mourner at a funeral, and I certainly did feel very limp. She was wearing a white dress and had her hair loose. I told her she looked quite ravishing like that.[15]

Mood is fragmented. There are sensations, images, and thoughts but no integration. The components are not functioning as a cohesive unit.

Sometimes people exaggerate or prolong one emotion. Actually they, too, must minimize some other emotion (since the total time in the day remains fixed). Consider learned sex-role stereotypes. Many men act strong and tough; they have learned to suppress their fear, longing, and vulnerability. Many women cry when confronted; they have learned to mistrust their assertiveness and power.

Each person has characteristic traits, ways of expressing—or, rather, meddling with—emotions: allowing some, exaggerating others, restraining others, detaching from still others. For example, some people habitually contain aggression, letting it out only as whimpering or complaining. Character traits are, in a way, meta-emotions, that is, orientations toward emotion.

Constraint, detachment, and exaggeration of emotion are not just learned in childhood. They are actively maintained in adulthood. The component dimensions of moods show this clearly, starting with the musculoskeletal aspect. A person who is careful about anger may habitually clench the jaw, constraining a quick, full anger into a subdued, careful expression. One who cries rarely and has a fear of crying may actually have a stiff upper lip—not just metaphorically but physically.

Blurring their vision and hearing, individuals who are cautious about feeling vulnerable may simply not see the attempts of others who are trying to comfort them. These people mistake a supportive tone for a patronizing tone and respond with caution and withdrawal. Exaggerated attention to visual details actually mediates paranoia; the hypervigilant, wide-eyed search for details in the environment provides the clues that prove persecution. "If I don't keep looking, they'll get me," a paranoid man might say. But if he didn't keep looking, he wouldn't see so many reasons to think they were going to get him.

Thoughts often serve to constrain emotion: "It's all my fault" or "Don't be ungrateful." Sometimes our thoughts compel us to indulge certain moods: "Act like a man" or "If they have a Porsche, we need one, too." An overreliance on logic and rationality often occurs in alienation, complementing and maintaining the detachment from emotion.

Character traits, too, manifest in the component facets of emotions. Someone who suppresses vulnerable feelings in favor of confident, successful feelings often looks "puffed up" and superior and (in the interpersonal dimension) often controls the conversation.

◎ TREATMENT

An unusual prevalence of one mood or the absence of a certain mood may signal emotional disturbance. In the client's personal history and life situation, has the individual expressed the appropriate emotion? If not, therapy can focus on catharsis of emotion or on skill and comfort with emotion. Catharsis is vivid, exciting, and relieving. In primal therapy, one cathartic school, the therapy is structured to maximize the intensity of the recall of childhood pain, deprivation, and anger. After letting go of the pressure of undischarged pain, the client is freer to get on with living in the present and planning the future.

By contrast, if the therapist focuses on facility with emotion, the client still recalls and ventilates past hurts, but the therapist makes no systematic attempt to ferret out all important traumata. Rather, the therapist helps the client become comfortable with moods. Future stress can then be discharged emotionally. As for past traumata, they are now more tolerable to the client as they arise in memory, so they gradually dissipate over time.

Catharsis makes a more vivid and dramatic therapy, but cultivation of the client's comfort and facility with emotions is more holistic. The client depends less on the therapist. To the extent that a person becomes more skillful at expressing anger in the presence of others, for example, he or she is more able to manage life on his or her own. Many clients complain today that they hear "take responsibility for your health" as a rebuke. They are not told how. By learning to express emotion, they can handle stress responsibly by ventilating it skillfully.

Many therapists encourage catharsis early in psychotherapy both to relieve tension and preoccupation enough to allow the client to pay attention with comfort and curiosity and also to give the client experience with intense emotion. Through catharsis, the client discovers directly that intense emotion is not an enemy but an ally. The emotion brings release. As therapy progresses over time, the focus shifts increasingly to the client's ability to express emotion. Having experienced emotion, the client then knows what to look for.

The practice with emotion can be structured or not. Assertiveness training, for example, uses certain standardized exercises for all clients. Gestalt therapists, by contrast, enter sessions without a planned program. They improvise experiments to highlight and amplify whatever the client feels that day. The client feels the mood, uses imagery to picture the context, and experiments with expressing the mood to the other people in the image. In a still less structured approach, some therapists simply encourage awareness of emotion and of inhibition of emotion. Without using exercises or experiments, they focus on the gradual cultivation of ease in emotion. Emotional therapy also need not even be explicit. The therapist may ask about events of daily life and say, for example, "How did the meeting go with your boss?" The session overtly centers on events, but the client's feelings about the events come out, too.

A method that emphasizes the client's ability to express emotion takes some time. It is easier to ventilate emotion than to learn such subtleties as assertiveness, tact, and discretion. On the job, we cannot usually say just how we feel. Further, many people certainly do deride or turn away from intimate expression, so being vulnerable is not safe with all of our acquaintances. Thus, after regaining the ability to express emotion, the client must still learn to choose the right time and place.

Often clients cannot practice expressing their emotion for they do not know what they feel. In *The Stranger*, Camus depicts a man who notices no emotion at all at the death of his mother—nor, it turns out, in most other events of his life:

Celeste was at his usual place beside the entrance, with his apron bulging on his paunch, his white mustache well to the fore. When he saw me he was sympathetic and 'hoped I wasn't feeling too badly.' I said, 'No,' but I was extremely hungry.[16]

In such cases of alienation, treatment must address not constraint of expression but rather lack of awareness of emotion. The emotional whole is fragmented. The therapist must repeatedly help the client notice the mood of the detached components: Behind aching shoulders the client may discover a feeling of shouldering burden; behind a red face, embarrassment.

A young teacher repeatedly complained that her awareness would become foggy just as she tried to address a difficult issue. She was annoyed at the fogginess and wanted it to go away. Encouraged to examine fogginess as a mood, she suddenly noticed that she did not want to continue when she felt foggy. The topic she was explaining had started to overwhelm her. She did not want to notice any more, so her awareness blurred.

A musician visited a neurologist repeatedly for hyperventilation. He would awaken at night breathing fast, his hands and lips numb and tingling. This hyperventilation syndrome, which occurs when one breathes deeply, disappears when one includes emotion with the exhalation: a sob, a curse, a cry of joy. In therapy, the musician imagined himself lying in bed, again breathing fast. Images of his mother arose. She was in the hospital, and he was afraid she was dying. The next day, he told his wife of his fear. She comforted him, and the hyperventilation did not return.

FROM OTHER DIMENSIONS TO EMOTIONS

Since mood is linked with other dimensions, practitioners can take emotional change as their goal, while investigating and intervening through other dimensions. In structural integration, or rolfing, the therapist uses deep massage of the muscles and their fascial covering to re-align the posture. But rolfers consider themselves more than masseurs. They emphasize that emotional scars heal and attitudes change through their work.

A family therapist often restructures the family system, for example, shifting an allegiance between mother and daughter to an alliance between mother and father. The problem under treatment may have been the daughter's anorexia nervosa (self-starvation) or her schizophrenia. So a social or interpersonal intervention may be an excellent treatment for an emotional problem.

Jogging often helps cure depression. If there is pent-up grief, allowing the chest to drop in exhalation can release it. Singing or shouting (common interventions to increase energy) can restore exuberance. Replacing self-deprecating thoughts with confident ones often works, too.

Is one component dimension best for approaching emotional problems? Sometimes for the anxious client who is hypoglycemic, for example, a low-sugar diet works more quickly and cheaply than dream exploration. More often, any dimension will do. Though Jungians favor symbols, Reichians body structure and energy, and Freudians transference (which occurs in the interpersonal dimension), a mood normally manifests in all these dimensions, and more, simultaneously.

A tentative way of walking into the room, a dream of being chased, shallow breathing, a sidelong glance in the session, or a strained tone of voice—any of these can tell the therapist to investigate, say, wariness. Further, the therapist can make interventions through any component dimension: "Walk around the office and stomp as you go" or "The next time you have that dream, turn and face the man who is chasing you" or "Breathe deeply" or "Look straight at me" or "Shout!"

Even the simplest encouragement to continue in the session broadens when the therapist takes a multidimensional perspective. A traditional verbal psychotherapist might say, "What are you thinking?" when the client pauses. A holistic therapist also might say, "What are you thinking?" but might equally say, "How does your body feel?" or "Are any images coming to you?" The therapist can even give a choice: "Check your body, your images, your vision, your sense of me. See what's coming up in any of those areas."

A shy, young woman in weekly psychotherapy falls silent for several minutes at the beginning of a session. Her lips are pressed together, her brow furrowed, her arms folded across her chest. The therapist finds himself picturing a schoolgirl sitting by herself in a long, high school corridor. Instinctively keeping away from her, other students talk in groups 30 feet down the hall.

Therapist: What's going on?
Client: I don't know.
T: How're you feeling right now?
C: Something's going on. I don't know what.
T: You look, maybe, angry to me and pushing it away.
C: Yeah? Maybe. But I don't know what at.
T: Watch your imagery.

C: Nothing's there.

T: Wait longer. Close your eyes and watch. Don't search, but be open to any picture. Describe whatever you see.

C: (Pause) I don't see much.

T: Let's take whatever comes. What's the not much?

C: I see a lake.

T: Describe it.

C: It's green. Kind of the color of the trees around. . . .

T: Keep going. Describe whatever you see.

C: Well, there are houses on the other side. It's this lake I went to with friends this weekend. I didn't have a very good time.

T: Oh?

C: Well I was bitchy the whole time. And I even told my girlfriend as we were driving up that I was bitchy, but she said, 'Don't be that way; have a good time.'

T: That's hard.

C: Yeah. I can't just stop being angry, but I feel like I'm supposed to. . . .

◎ FROM EMOTION TO OTHER DIMENSIONS

Treating emotional problems successfully will simultaneously improve linked or component dimensions. When a man has tensed neck or belly muscles to restrain anger, headaches disappear and constipation and peptic ulcers abate as he becomes comfortable with anger. His dancing may change from rigid to inspired as he becomes willing to "be moved." For the woman who has fragmented emotion into isolated components, images, thoughts, and sensations begin to make sense as emotion becomes tolerable. She may realize that one friend is a pain in the neck and another makes her sick and tired. She will expect a war dream, but not fear it, when she goes to bed angry.

Even diet may improve. A young woman told of a repetitious, years-long cycle of dieting and successfully losing 20 pounds, only to regain the weight as soon as she had reached her ideal shape. Encouraged to imagine herself dieting and then to focus on her mood, she noticed a strong competitiveness. Next, she stood up and walked around the room, imagining herself slender. She felt calm and gentle, but she missed her competitiveness. Now, her cycles of dieting and weight gain made sense. In order to express her competitiveness in the realm of weight, she had to be losing weight actively, so she had to be overweight. At her ideal weight, she had no outlet for her competitiveness. So she decided to shift the arena of competition. She successfully pursued a man she wanted to win, and she worked to become top salesperson in her firm. Her weight stabilized.

Fuller emotion—combined with self-knowledge and discretion—raises the quality of life. It brings passion, exuberance, and fire. When we are not overwhelmed by moods, we can be compassionate to others and not back off when they are full of feeling. We can resonate with them and be close.

Finally, as we watch emotions to learn about them, awareness benefits. To the extent that we habitually constrain or avoid feeling certain emotions, we do not prevent the moods, we simply have diminished awareness while in those moods. In meditation, we can allow awareness to move spontaneously from the breath to the body to thoughts to intentions and to moods. As we practice meditation, we become mindful an increasing percentage of the time. In order to be mindful, we must accept and stay with all the experiences that awareness touches. Emotions are quite difficult to watch in this relaxed, curious way. We either dislike them and want them to go away or we like them and, with little awareness, try to keep them around. To watch them without being carried away cultivates a certain rigor of mindfulness, an impeccability.[17, 18]

Perhaps the spiritual path and the emotional path can be reconciled. In being spiritual, we aspire to be free from greed, anger, and suffering. But that is a goal. Along the way, we still have emotions. To expect freedom from emotion simply by wishing strongly enough leads only to guilt and self-criticism. Seeing dark moods clearly, we do not want to prolong them. Seeing our context, our effect on others, we want to express just enough, not to exaggerate the moods and cause pain, guilt, or reprisal. And with long, careful play with emotion, we can sometimes catch a mood so close to its arising that mindfulness itself restores equilibrium. Then, effortlessly and without suppression, emotions come and go, and awareness remains clear. The upward-bound traveler and the downward-bound traveler can pause together, exchange information, and help each other.

REFERENCES

1. J. Needleman, Talk delivered in a conference at the C.G. Jung Institute of San Francisco, 1975.

2. Lowell Cohn, "Al Attles is Too Nice," *San Francisco Chronicle*, Monday Feb. 2, 1981.

3. Jean-Paul Sartre, *Nausea*. (New York: New Directions, 1964).

4. Anagarika Munindraji, Personal communication.

5. Joseph Goldstein, Dharma talk, Yucca Valley, 1981.

6. Martin Heidegger, *Being and Time* (New York: Harper & Row, 1962).

7. Eugene T. Gendlin, "Befindlischkeit: Heidegger and the Philosophy of Psychology," *Review of Existential Psychology and Psychiatry*, XVI (1978): 43–71.

8. Heidegger, *Being and Time*, p. 142.

9. *Ibid.*, p. 339.

10. William Gass, *On Being Blue, A Philosophical Inquiry* (Boston: Godine, 1976), p. 78.

11. *Ibid.*, p. 53.

12. Paul Ekman and Wallace Friesen, *Unmasking the Face* (Englewood Cliffs, N.J.: Prentice-Hall, 1975).

13. Albert Camus, *The Stranger* (New York: Vintage, 1954), p. 53.

14. *Ibid.*, p. 50.

15. *Ibid.*, p. 59.

16. *Ibid.*, p. 31.

17. Joseph Goldstein, *The Experience of Insight* (Santa Cruz: Unity Press, 1976).

18. Carlos Casteneda, *The Teachings of Don Juan* (New York: Simon and Schuster, 1969).

11

THE SYMBOLIC DIMENSION

ALBERT KREINHEDER, Ph.D.

My own experience with rheumatoid arthritis is an example of symbolic healing. Before the arthritis, I was a typically healthy person, with only minor exceptions. If illness came, I just waited for three days, and my condition improved. Or I went to the doctor, he gave me a pill, and before long, I was well again. On the whole, I convinced myself that my body had become invincible—at least for 30 more years.

It was, incongruously, at a time I thought my health to be superb that arthritis visited me. I had been running four miles a day, but now after only two hours of being awake each morning, I needed to withdraw to bed to recover my strength. The pain progressed through my body. First, my hip wouldn't work. Then my knees, ankles, toes, and fingers would not work. I had great difficulty walking, and it was almost impossible to get up from a chair or to sit down again once I was up. The worst of it was that my bodily state had, I suspected, some kind of connection or relationship to my total personality. Wasn't I, despite my pretense of openness and liberality, a rather rigid and constricted person?

Yet, as my joints were growing stiffer and more inflamed, a strange thing was happening. I was dreaming of warm, sensuous women. In my quiet hours when I turned inward, I heard sometimes the soft voice of a lovely woman. I spoke to her. Day after day, I carried on dialogues with her in my imagination, and I carefully recorded them in writing. Our relationship grew, in time, to be intensely personal and intimate. Although this was, strictly speaking, all in my imagination, it seemed absolutely real—more so than anything else I had going at the time. Without a doubt, it eventually helped to produce substantial changes in my personality, including my body. From my closeness to her, I learned how starved I was for affection.

Paradoxically, while I was frozen in my joints, humiliated by my neurosis, and sicker than ever, she was coming to me more vividly and dramatically. She brought exactly what I needed: softness, suppleness, capriciousness, a delightful variety and animation—the very things I had suppressed during my long drive for achievement. As I reached for her, she too was reaching for me, not because we were so alike but rather because there was such a polarity. We each had what the other needed. It was hard for me to see what she needed from me, but she did need me. Only through me could she actualize herself, and that became very important to her.

"Oh," I complained to her, "how my bones are aching. Please, can't you come and warm me with your body heat? I am so weak and empty. How I need you now."

I had learned that I must ask for what I need. That is the first step. But did I even know what I needed? All my life, I had been fearful and tense, trying too hard, always alert, vigilant, and competitive. I knew certainly that I did not need all that, but what did I need? I needed her, but I wasn't sure exactly why; I simply craved her.

She told me not to worry. "If you ask for me, I come. I live. I am. My name is Love. It is I you need and wish for. Just ask for me. I'll come."

At last I knew her name: Love. That's what I needed. Love was the oil that would lubricate my aching joints.

"Just ask," she said. "I'll come. My love will enter you in every part."

"Will you enter where it hurts? Will you warm my hand, my elbow, and my rusty hips?" I asked.

"I will. But in those places where you are afraid of love, I cannot enter. Release those parts to me; then all will soon be well again."

But I could not yield that readily. It would take time. I had an image of what to do, but I couldn't do it yet. The arthritis was still getting worse. Yet I was growing closer to this imaginary woman, and my hopeful expectations were increasing.

"Come," I called to her. "Repair my wounds. Loosen my joints. Break through the fear, and soothe me with your love so we may move in unison, you and I together."

"I am here," she said, "to wake you from your frozen sleep. Come alive. Run, swim, dance, laugh, move, shout, and play. Your strain and stiffness need not be. Cast off those fetters, breathe, relax. Be full and move with me. It is easy now that I am with you."

Her words affected me, but I was no better. It would be eight months before the symptoms would ease. The impact of her love would have its effect; but, for now, I needed lots and lots of softening. In some way, too, I still needed the suffering and the disability. It was my ordeal of fire, a contrast or backdrop against which her appearances were more dramatic and appreciated.

Two months passed, and the pain was getting worse. In every joint of my body, it felt like the dry bones were grating against each other. I wanted to be emotionally fluid and glistening like Love, but I was still far from it. It seemed that I needed the disease to convince me how petrified and obstinate I had become. I was acutely aware of my need, and I knew at last what to ask for.

I thought of the full, round nudes of Renoir; how replenishing it would be to have contact with such a fresh, succulent body. Renoir must also have been desiccated within to have sought out such plump forms. I told my friend Love again about my pain and the dry bones, and I asked her for the gift of moisture.

"I will feed your body with my fluids," she replied. "Touch my wetness. I bring forth the slippery waters, opening the path of love. Hold me and be with me in the waters."

Despite this rejuvenating influence, I still felt locked into my rigidities, as if I had to experience fully just how immobile I had become. With her I could be friendly and warm, but out in the world, I was formal and impersonal, especially with strangers. I approached them like potential enemies with my armor on and swords ready. Unfortunately, such a fearful, tightly guarded posture hardly projected a picture of strength.

One morning when traveling, I left my motel room and was greeted by a robust man who smiled broadly, "I'm Jim Sanders. I'm sure glad to meet you!" I looked at him as if a tarantula had walked across my path, and I refused to shake his hand. He shrugged. "That's what's wrong with the world. Nobody cares about anyone else anymore."

Then I remembered Love. I looked at the man and saw perplexity and disappointment in him. I apologized. It felt good to humble myself, to feel a little current of warmth flow through me. He forgave me instantly and told me that he was on his way to put flowers on his father's grave. "I just discovered that I really loved the old man, and now I want to tell everyone about it."

Perhaps it's better to be detained occasionally—to be bored, even swindled, once in a while than to lose out totally on the chance for intimacy with another person. I had been dealing with people as if they were vending machines. You put in a quarter, pull the right levers, and something comes back. But that's not a relationship; it's a transaction—neat, fast, clearcut. Don't mess up your life with crazy people and their problems. Don't smile, you will look like an idiot.

I told all this to Love. I was bringing everything to her now, especially the deepest and most agitating things.

"Yes, you certainly do have a brutal, stiff, unyielding attitude," she said, "but not toward me because now you have softened in your love and trust of me. At last, you feel a horror at that wall you have against the world. Let us tear down the wall together."

"Someday," she continued, "you will cry, and when you dissolve into tears, you will be loose again. Once there was no wall. Once you were not stiff. You cried. You shouted. You were a supple child. Give in to your weakness. Be ill. Be helpless. It does not matter now. Be what you are. Don't hide your weakness with a grim, determined face. Cry, moan, stumble, let it show. Believe in your gifts, for they are good. Do not try to make them other than what they are. Be free and do not strive. I live like that, and I am content, quiet in myself, and moving free."

The pain continued to spread. It was everywhere now, in my

back, knees, hips, chest, toes and ankles, even in my jawbone. I observed it. I lived with it. I watched it curiously. It loomed up before me as the biggest thing in my life. There we were, me and the pain. One sleepless night when I lay writhing in its grip, pain seemed to me like an entity in itself, some tormenting incubus. I decided to speak to it:

Me: You hold me tight in your grip and do not let me go. If you crave my undivided attention, you have received it. Whatever I attend to, I must also attend to you. Even when I write, I feel you in my hand, in all parts of my body. I am terribly frightened of you. Why are you here?

Pain: I am here to get your attention, to make known my presence. I have a power beyond your power. My will surpasses yours. You cannot prevail over me, but I can easily prevail over you.

Me: But why must you show me this power and destroy me with it?

Pain: I show you because I will no longer let you disregard me. You can no longer treat me as if I am not. You will know my power, and you will humble yourself before me. I am the first of all things, and all things spring from me; without me there is nothing. I crave your attention. I want you to see me and feel me and hear me and bring to me the best of yourself. I want to be with you closely in your thoughts at all times. That is why I make you think only of me. Now, with my presence in you, you can no longer live the same way and do the same things. You cannot use your mind in the old ways, for now you must give yourself only to contemplation of me. But out of this will come many good things.

This encounter with my pain marked a turning point. Now I had a meaning to the pain, a plan to follow, a responsibility, someone who cared.

Until the time of my sickness, I had thought of myself as a person strongly committed to growth and greater consciousness. But I was realizing how inert we humans are. Before doing anything really radical about ourselves, we have to be driven to desperation. Something had to be very wrong for me to be as sick as I was. So, to get it right again, big changes would have to be made. The sickness was not really the sickness at all. It was the cure. We are sick in our minds, sick in our lives, sick in our values and in our behavior. Physical symptoms prod us to change our ways, urging us to be well again in our total selves. The so-called sickness is the entry of the curative factor.

I could stand the pain. What was worse was the fear that accompanied it. Was my body deteriorating? Was death close at hand? If so, I was not ready. I had to get my life in order, bring it to a graceful completion, be at last a whole person. Out of my fear came the thought that my body was like my mother's body, weak and susceptible to illness. Then, more irrationally, I thought that my body actually was her body. When that seemed impossible, I thought, "Ah, the body is really the living concrete existence in us of the great mother goddess, the *Magna Mater*, the *mater*ial part of ourselves." Fantastic idea, but one I willingly believed, and out of my belief, I prayed to the great mother goddess. And, through my prayers, I felt more than ever that she was always with me and so close to me that she literally was my body. When I asked her who she was, she said, "I am the basis and the bottom of your life and your beginning. Your body still is mine, as it always was. Love me in your body, and in your body worship me."

I stopped worrying about being vain or narcissistic and just gloried in how beautiful my body was. Then came a gentle, soothing energy through my body that seemed incompatible with any illness. I dove into a swimming pool. I made tentative over-arm strokes with no pain in my shoulders. My limbs moved freely and loosely. I was bursting with gratitude and disbelief—it had happened! The arthritis was not all gone in a day, but from that swim forward, I began to heal. "Thank you, thank you," I murmured. How precious a gift! Yet, it had taken much time and devoted effort to make myself ready to receive the gift.

◎ THE SYMBOLIC CONTENT OF ILLNESS

In my occupation with the subject of healing, I became aware that every pain, every illness, every symptom, has a psychological content. This is the symbolic part. This is the way the imagination perceives the illness or the symptom. For example, when I talked to my arthritis pain, my imagination perceived the pain as a demon or god who desired intimacy with me. Presumably, as our intimacy increased, he would be less inclined to torture me with pain.

The symbolic content may be difficult to capture but, nevertheless, it is always there. Though it is gone now, I had, for some time after my arthritis was healed, a residual pain and weakness in my left foot. I want to illustrate how I got hold of the symbolic content behind that pain:

Again, I used a figure who came to me in dream and fantasy. He was a medical doctor and psychotherapist named Kieffer, who appeared to me in a dream. We had many conversations on illness and healing. Through this dialogue, I gathered much of my understanding of healing.

I told him about the lingering problem with my left foot, explaining that I was doing everything I could—massaging it, exercising it, pushing it to harder usage.

"You do all those practical things, of course," he said, "but the real issue is with the symbols. What about your foot? What image does it raise in your mind? Can you tell me that?"

"Well, yes," I replied. "I see an old man hobbling with a cane. He's not troubled very much by the lame foot. His attention is on other things."

"What things? What kind of person is he?"

"He's very alive mentally. I suppose you might say he is a deep person, religious maybe, a kind of philosopher. He is like a wise teacher. People come to him because he inspires them and gives them insight."

"So," replied Kieffer, "you see. All *that* is centered in your bad foot. It's really non-essential whether the foot gets better or not. That will take care of itself because it's really not the problem. The problem is that you have been unaware of the interesting old man. Perhaps the foot trouble is there so that you will limp a little, so that you will get a feeling of his presence, and even for a time, feel a bit like him yourself. His presence will probably change you quite a bit. You see, when you stop cursing the symptoms and get deeper into the images instead, then the healing comes. But the healing never starts at the place of the symptom. Your foot doesn't get better. Maybe later it will, but not as the first thing. First you have to be healed in your soul."

"Every illness," he explained, "is an onslaught upon the person as he or she is. Things have become so bad, and the person is so alienated from the whole of life, that an extreme invasion is necessary to break into the hardened formation of the person. An individual must be weakened and crushed so that he or she will finally be so loosened and liquefied that the life spirit can flow in. To be sick is to be shut off, to be isolated. Every disease is like an invading force trying to destroy our rigid forms and make us whole. With every invading illness, there comes also a symbolic content, and it is the task of the soul to expand itself so that it can encompass the invading images and symbols. This may, at first, be a struggle, but ultimately, it becomes an expansive, releasing process as one grows beyond his or her former boundaries.

"The disease won't let us live the old way," he continued. "It actually comes to destroy the way we are. The stiffness in your movements is due to the way you have held yourself. It is from a guarded, fearful, cautious posture, a carefulness to control tears, blushing, and anger, and free, spontaneous movements. The symptoms are the crying out of the body telling you it has had enough. The symptoms will tear you apart at the very places where you have held too tightly."

"But sometimes," I said, "it all seems to be more than I can cope with."

"You may think so but not really," he said. "We never get more than we can handle. Even if it means death. Death can be handled. The object of healing is not to stay alive. It is to move closer to wholeness. Healing may take place in death; death is the final healing. Whatever comes is ours, and we can handle it.

"When we become ill, it is as if we have been chosen or elected, not to be limited and crippled, but to be healed. The disease always carries its own cure and also the cure for our whole personality. If we take it as our own and stay with this new experience, with the pain and the fear and all the accompanying images, we will be healed to a wholeness far beyond our previous so-called health."

He said further, "I'm not talking about simple headaches and stomachaches and such things. They could be just the result of wrong living and can easily be remedied. I'm talking about the big, overwhelming diseases that come like a bolt from the blue. An outside force comes with no seeming logic whatsoever. Then one curses God and asks, 'Why me?' That's a rational question asked as if there ought to be a cause and effect, as if we did something wrong, and now this horrible consequence comes. Perhaps it is in one's fate. God does not punish us. He selects us."

I told Kieffer he was confusing me.

"Of course, because we are getting into the irrational," he said. "When we come up against an unknowable power, when we can't explain something, then there is a terrible fear. It's absolutely awesome to be struck by a serious disease. And the images that come with the disease will be just as awesome. In order to deal with them, the more irrational you are, the better. Just think the craziest thoughts you are capable of, ideas like your mother pulling you into her grave, and then you're on the right track. For God's sake, just don't try to be logical about it. If you can live with the ghosts and the other weird and monstrous things, then you have a chance to be healed."

"But," I queried, "how can I ever live with things like that?"

"You can't, of course, but they are there. They make your hair stand on end. And if they do touch you, their power gets into you. That's the life power. That's what heals. It gets into you, and your body comes alive."

◎ THE LIFE POWER

That power, that life power, became very important to me. It seemed like the whole essence of healing. It was, for me, the ultimate kind of benefit to be obtained from the symbolic mode of healing. The power is a tangible energy that comes as a physical sensation along with the involvement with symbols. Under the right conditions, certain experiences provoked in me a definite physical response. Although there had been no contact with another object or person, no drug, no agent other than the pure psychological process of imagining, there were definite bodily reactions. It was like a heat or a chill, a tingling, a creeping of the flesh. When these sensations occurred, the experience for me was of my body being entered by some outside force, not merely by an energy but by a being of some sort—an intelligence. And that intelligence, that being, was aware that I was aware of it.

At first, these experiences filled me with an unearthly fear, especially when they came unexpectedly, as when I awoke with night terrors, hyperventilating, with panic in my breast. But even in the best of circumstances, the power is always awesome and uncanny. Though it may touch us lightly and benignly, it is an invisible presence beyond our understanding.

It appeared to me also that illness comes when this life power invades our body, and we are unable to accommodate it. Whether the energy was helpful or destructive seemed to depend upon whether or not it could be contained in our consciousness and harmonized with our conscious point of view. Can we feel its presence, accept it, acknowledge it, hold it within our perception, actually feel ourselves to be in relation to it? Then it is the symbolic entity we long for but fear in his coming. How we crave his coming. How gentle and terrible he is, like liquid fire, but also like the soothing hands of a beloved friend.

To receive the power and to hold it in quiet stillness is a joyful experience, as if one is totally and absolutely loved. The power will be benevolent and not destructive if we are able to achieve a loving relationship with it. This may come only after extensive encounters with a symbolic figure in our imagery. For me, my relationship with the woman as an inner symbol was very important, as I needed first to acquire through her influence more erotic sensibility, more warmth, more ability to reach out to others and to care about them. A head-on collision with the power without the mediating agency of love can be disastrous. Once, in a dream, I actually saw the power. It stood like a wall of quivering lightning 10 feet away from me. But between me and the power was the woman, and she protected me from it.

The awareness of the power is central to the symbolic experience. Unless this bodily component is present, we are not yet reaching fully into our symbols. True imagination is never just in the head. It is also in the body, including all those peculiar radiating sensations I have described. That is why, when we finally achieve the symbolic life, we feel it from head to toe, and there are observable physical effects. We are no longer the same person as before. We actually look different; our friends no longer respond to us in the same way.

◎ SIGNS, SYMBOLS, AND PERSONAL SYMBOLS

What exactly are symbols? A symbol, first of all, is different from a sign. A sign is a representation by word or picture or diagram of something that actually exists objectively and is tangibly visible to all observers. Thus, the word "chair" is a sign for the thing "chair." Symbols, on the other hand, point to things that are mysterious and ultimately unknowable but which are, nevertheless, known to exist because of observable effects they have. One of the effects is the symbols themselves. They spring into our perception full born and, if we let them touch us at all, they touch us deeply and in a different place than do ordinary events. My own symbolic experience happens specifically with *my own* personal symbols. They are living symbols because they live in me. It is *my* symbolic experience because it raises the hair on my neck. It may happen in reading a poem, in finding a stone on the beach, in focusing intently upon a dream image. It is the numinous experience. It is a theophany, a showing forth of the god power. It requires no religious faith, just receptiveness to our inner experience and willingness to take it seriously.

A symbol is both rational and irrational, having some appeal to our logical understanding but also being mysterious and unfathomable. It is physical but also psychological. It is delicate and woven fine like a fleeting phantasm, yet it also has real substance. The miracle of the symbolic experience is that, when we are in the symbolic mode with the images in focus and the strange sensations in the body, we are at that moment completely whole. And if we were but able to achieve that state regularly, we would more surely come to a consistent inner wholeness and the eventual healing of our ills.

◎ THE SYMBOLIC MODE OF TREATMENT

In my role as psychotherapist, I consistently use the symbolic mode of treatment, but I doubt whether it should be systematized into a formal method that can be learned by practitioners and then applied. It seems wiser that the therapist's training for this approach consist primarily of his or her own extensive engagements with symbolic images. Then the therapist will probably not pursue any clearcut method or treatment plan but rather will be sensitive to those symbols which arise from the psyche of the client. The therapist will support those modes of relating to the symbols that spring naturally from the growth movements within the client. This would be highly individual, and hardly ever will any two cases be alike.

The personality of the therapist is of much greater importance than the armamentarium of techniques, though the therapist certainly ought to know, on theoretical grounds, what he or she is doing. As one who evokes the life power in others, the therapist will be most effective if the power is alive in him or her. When, in the analytical hour, the therapist feels the power within, the chilling tingle in the spine, the warm current moving through the body, then the power has come. Then the therapist may give silent thanks, for healing is under way.

An underlying assumption of this work is that there is a dynamism within the individual that is reaching toward wholeness. The dreams and the spontaneous imagination compensate for the limited viewpoint of consciousness. It is as if they say, "See here, don't you think you ought to pay attention to these issues?" The human organism strives for equilibrium and completeness. Dreams, because they correct the one-sided conscious position, always bring us exactly what is most needed. Unfortunately, the conscious mind, if it listens at all, is apt to distort the meaning of the dream to fit its own prejudices. How beneficial it is to walk around imaginatively inside of the dream, accepting all its premises with an absolute belief in the reality of the world we have entered! Then it is as if we are washed clean of fixed patterns and given a bath of renewal in the larger psyche.

When we enter the world of dream and symbol, there is an interface of the conscious mind with the unconscious, particularly when we converse directly with dream figures. These inner personalities seem to operate quite independently of any conscious direction. Once we are able to let them speak without trying to direct them, we are genuinely surprised at what comes out. Then we have the secret, joyful knowledge that there is life in us; there are dimensions of our being of which we never knew before.

The realm of the image figures was called by C. G. Jung the *objective psyche* to emphasize that the images are not thought up by the person but seem, on the contrary, to be happening to him or her. When we go deep into our subjectivity, we discover a world of objects, a moving drama that we ourselves do not create. In our habitually outward-oriented stance, we are totally oblivious to this inner drama. If it does leak through in sleep or in some other altered state, we immediately rationalize it away. If it penetrates more forcibly as in a nightmare, we quickly turn on the light, and assure ourselves that it was nothing but a dream.

Often, there is a stubborn unwillingness to venture into the shadowy world of symbols. This reluctance should be accepted by the therapist, for he or she must not enter before the client is ready. The readiness will increase as the personality strengthens, so preliminary work to that end is advisable—helping the client let go of hang-ups, see personal "scripts," express emotions, and open up anxieties. When the client is stronger, he or she will be curious and interested in the symbolic world. Then, the time is right.

When we begin the symbolic work, it is important to engage actively and not merely enjoy fantasies in a passive way. Some people are already too immersed in their drowsy dream world. Others like to astonish the therapist with their virtuosity in the creation of images. They can easily take off on dizzy flights of fancy that have no connection with themselves in their real life. The most effective imagination is a dialogue with the dream figures. In doing this, the person stays oriented to his or her personal point of view, interests, needs, and personal problems, and expresses them while remaining open to new information from the symbolic figure. This results in an encounter, a negotiation, a mutual understanding, a coming to terms. In this way, conscious and unconscious make a bridge to each other, and in their meeting, a new center is formed to a now-enlarged personality.

This active interaction between ego and the unconscious is the gist of the symbolic mode of healing. If the ego is too passive, there can be an over-dominance of the unconscious with a consequent weakening of the ego. The ego can then be flooded with images and impulses that may impell it to inappropriate behavior. Moodiness is a prime example: either those dark moods of total unworthiness or, perhaps, an inflated sense of "god almightiness" where we feel ourselves to be as omnipotent and as all-knowing as the soaring imagination will allow. At the extreme is the full-blown psychotic, who takes the irrationality of the dream world as everyday reality. Obviously, in this kind of therapy, guidance is essential, and people with unformed egos should stay away from it altogether.

As is always asked with every kind of therapy, "When am I ready to leave the therapist and go out on my own?" The client is ready when he or she is able to work independently. This means that the client has learned to avoid all the pitfalls of imagination and also has developed a point of reference outside the self. When able to sustain no dialogue other than the ego talking to the ego, the client is still stewing in his or her own juice without an outside viewpoint. The client is probably then, as often happens when engaged in "self-analysis," merely strengthening and reinforcing neurosis, for there is no input other than the one-sided view of the conscious self.

The therapist's role, in this case, is to serve as an advocate of the unconscious, interpreting its position in an attempt to challenge the client. When the client can listen to and heed the voice of the unconscious, the voice of the symbolic image figure; can dialogue with it; and can contain the life power that runs through the body whenever he or she is intimately involved with inner symbols, then the client has found the way to wholeness. The client has found a healer who is nearer than his or her own heart.

12

THE SENSORY/ IMAGERY DIMENSION

EMMETT M. MILLER, M.D.

We take in the environment through our senses: vision, hearing, smell, taste, and touch. Our senses give us information, and they shape our intellect and our choices. They influence our actions and our interactions. The senses normally give us accurate and relevant feedback about the environment. Pleasure in a sensation tells us to remain or to return. Pain tells us to leave or to avoid the situation in the future. After working for hours, for example, we may begin to have tension in the muscles of the shoulders and back. Sensing this discomfort, we take a rest. Pain, at times, demands our creativity and even inspires our personal growth.

Structural malformations and neurological diseases only rarely impair sensory perception. Most often, diminished perception of sensory input results from chronic inattention to sensory media. At a boring lecture, we notice the uncomfortable chair and the stuffy room; at an interesting presentation, we do not. The same percepts are there, but we ignore them. This inattention can quite quickly shut off valuable sensory input. As an experiment, make a fist and hold it tightly for three or four minutes. You will notice a sensation of discomfort and pain that gradually turns into a feeling of tingling. Finally, you will experience a feeling of numbness and an actual decrease in the sensation coming from the tightened fist. The same chain of events happens when we work and feel the tension in the shoulder and back muscles and do not respond to the tension but rather continue to work on in the same way. Our senses eventually cease giving data about the increased tension. We lose our signal to relax, and the tension and spasm of the muscles continue and can even deteriorate into symptoms and structural pathology.

Some individuals, popularly termed "negative," selectively focus upon the unpleasant sensations in life. They feel the pain and the excessive heat of the environment. On a partly sunny day, they notice the clouds. This bias in sensory perception produces depression and hopelessness and detracts from happiness and motivation. Likewise, there are those who see only the rosy side of life. They are seldom prepared for the harsh realities.

◎ IMAGERY

So, through our senses, we perceive the environment. In all five senses, we can also imagine the world when no corresponding object is present. This mental imagery can be nearly as vivid and compelling to the senses as perception. Try the following exercise. First, read the following paragraph. Then close your eyes, and carry out the instructions in imagery.

Imagine that, in your hand, you have a ripe, yellow lemon. Feel the roughness of the skin of the lemon and the firmness of its surface. Imagine that, in your other hand, you have a shiny, sharp, stainless steel knife. Imagine placing the lemon on a cutting board and, using the knife, neatly slicing it in half. See the drops of lemon juice on the shiny surface of the blade. See the cut halves of the lemon—their shininess. See the sections of the lemon—the seeds that have been cut in half. Imagine now that you're taking one of these halves and squeezing the juice into a sparkling clean, empty glass. Using both of your hands, squeeze as much juice out of this half a lemon as you can. Now picture bringing the glass up to your lips. See the yellow lemon juice in the bottom of the glass. Smell the strong odor of lemons as you bring it close to your nose. Tip the glass so that the lemon juice flows into your mouth and over the surface and around the sides of your tongue. Taste the sour, acid flavor. Please stop reading at this point and carry out this exercise before continuing.

The lemon we imagine looks, smells, and tastes remarkably like lemons we have actually perceived. Memories of perceptions may be combined to create images never experienced before. We may never have cut a lemon with a shiny, stainless steel knife, but, if we have ever used a stainless steel knife and have experienced a cut lemon, we will be able to create this complex image. Our emotional and physical response to any given image is unique and is ultimately based upon previous experience. Some people eat lemons right out of the skin and enjoy them, for example, while others find they are far too sour. When most of us imagine the lemon in the exercise, we notice a markedly increased flow of saliva, a flow much the same as would have been generated had we tasted actual lemon juice and not just its image. Although an actual lemon would cause almost immediate salivation, at least several seconds are necessary to create a sufficiently clear image to produce the same response.

Imagery is most realistic and evokes the strongest physiological response when several senses are included. Also, previous experience is necessary for this integrative use of imagery; if we had never tasted a lemon or other citrus fruit, we would not respond to the imagery with salivation.

Very clear imagery is the rule rather than the exception in early childhood. For the young child, the lines between fantasy and reality are so thin that they constantly shift back and forth. Many children have make-believe playmates, which may be human or animal, that they can relate to completely. The ease with which children play pretend games, compared to the difficulty that most adults seem to have getting into these games, points up this fact. The increasing importance placed upon intellectual development (left-brain/linear, verbal processing skills) probably tends to reciprocally inhibit natural imagery, so adults have less comfort and facility with fantasy.

Everyone is capable of imaging, although some people naturally are more inclined to find it an easier task than others. Artists, designers, and craftspeople work with imagery all the time. The excited, high school basketball player may put himself to sleep each night picturing himself making baskets. The individual with stage fright may worry herself sick for weeks picturing her audience laughing at her. Mark Spitz, the Olympic swimmer, would imagine a beautiful girl at either end of the pool. The more beautiful she was, the faster he swam toward her.

The storage capacity for images is immense. Many people believe that every single experience is stored for the duration of an individual's life, though some images are more easily retrieved than others. Although each individual tends to be more familiar with using one internal representational system (auditory, visual, or kinesthetic), facility in the other two systems can easily be developed through practice. There are certain times when a person is more likely to experience clear and vivid imagery. Most people experience it during dreams, and during the period just before going to sleep or just after waking up. In hypnosis or in states of deep relaxation, imagery is usually quite vivid. After taking psychedelic drugs, such as LSD, psilocybin, or even marijuana, many people immediately experience images. During the relaxation following sexual orgasm, imagery is also spontaneous.

Imagery helps us take a number of possibilities and try them out in our imagination before selecting the one that will actually work in a given situation. For example, if we have a number of boards of various lengths and a stream across which we wish to build a bridge, we can look at each board and at the stream and, with imagery, determine which board is the proper length to go across the stream by picturing whether it would reach across or fall through. This gives us the ability to recombine past experiences in the thinking and reasoning processes.

Imagery is an indicator and determinant of emotional functioning. Imagining ourselves well-liked and cared for, we experience a simultaneous feeling of well-being. Imagining people plotting against us, we are much less emotionally secure. In physical function, our imagery often influences energy level and amount of tension carried in the body and contributes to such diseases as headaches, gastrointestinal disturbances, hypertension, and asthma.

◎ THE SELF-IMAGE

We see ourselves as individuals within a certain environment. The various characteristics ascribed to the individual vis-a-vis the environment make up the self-image: I am assertive, frightened, friendly, intelligent, lonely, likely to succeed. The self-image can be said to be functioning properly when it results in a sense of well-being associated with a healthy, balanced lifestyle. Positive self-image results in appropriate responses to realistic situations in the environment.

Maxwell Maltz describes individuals who underwent plastic surgery to correct disfiguring aspects of the face. Prior to surgery, their self-image was of being unattractive. Following plastic surgery, he noted that some people continued to act unattractive; they were shy and unwilling to be seen in public places. Even though their physical image had changed, their inner self-image had not. His approach was to work with the person on visualizing a more attractive inner self-image. This resulted in a disappearance of the shy behavior, and they were able to function better in the world.[1]

Carl Simonton, a physician working with cancer patients, gave tests to clients at the beginning of their treatment. As a result of the tests, he rated people as being extremely positive, positive-negative, and extremely negative. He found that those who had negative expectations and images about the treatment did actually succumb quickly to their disease, whereas the extremely positive group had quicker and longer remissions.[2] If a person makes a clear image of what he or she wants and motivates the mind toward that image, there will be a tendency for the unconscious parts of the mind to strive toward bringing that final, desired outcome to pass.

Imagery can be explicit or implicit. Most of the time, our imagery is implicit; that is, our behavior and response to ongoing situations occur as if we were behaving according to certain images, but we are not consciously aware of any specific imagery. Thus, several hours before giving a public talk, an individual may be frightened, have elevated blood pressure, be trembling, nervous, or emotionally distraught. Although there may be no image in awareness, if we ask this person to visualize himself during the talk, he will probably picture himself being laughed at, forgetting lines, and so forth. Similarly, if we are non-assertive, we behave as if following the image of being inferior to those around us. When asked to create a picture of what is going on internally, we might describe the friends as seeming much larger than us. Here, we have made explicit the implicit image of being inferior to friends. As an implicit image becomes explicit, therapeutic intervention usually becomes easier.

◎ ASSESSMENT

The practitioner can assess explicit experience with imagery by asking questions such as, "Do you ever sit and picture things; do you daydream and picture what is about to come? Do you find yourself forming images (auditory, visual, or kinesthetic) of upcoming events? Do you see images—positive or negative?"

Another, more subtle, way of assessing imaging ability, is to ask the person to picture the desired outcome. For instance, a person may express that he or she is experiencing too much stress and would like to have the stress level reduced. Ask the person how he or she would be different after stress is reduced. Suggest that the person look into the future as if watching a movie of himself or herself. Ask the person to describe how he or she would look after making the desired change. Have the person close his or her eyes and see how he or she would picture this.

The most direct way to test the person's ability to form images is to have him or her relax and imagine something pleasant and familiar. In general, imaging becomes easier, more vivid, and more effective if the person is in a relaxed state. Most practitioners who employ therapeutic imagery do so after inducing a deeply relaxed or hypnotic state in the client. This may be done by having the person first relax the toes, then the feet, the ankles, and so forth all the way up to the neck. Finally, the muscles of the face and those around the eyes are relaxed. This entire process might take from three to ten minutes, depending upon the person's initial level of tension and anxiety. When a person is relaxed, the body appears to be still, the eyes are usually closed, the eyelids sometimes flutter, and the person usually has a relaxed expression on his or her face.

After inducing this state of relaxation, the person is invited to choose a pleasant image to look at. The person may choose something from the distant past or something from present life, or he or she may look forward to the future. It is suggested that the person bring the image in clearly, seeing the colors, hearing the sounds, feeling the movement, and enjoying the sensations. The instructions are given slowly to give the individual an opportunity to assess the various sensations in the imagery. The person is then gradually returned to an awareness of his or her surroundings. Questions are asked about the type of images, their clarity, and the feelings that accompany them.

Aspects of self-image are ascertained with some degree of accuracy by having an individual picture himself or herself in a particular situation, that is, to imagine speaking in front of a group, going for a job interview, or some other situation that is pertinent to the individual's present-day life. If a person is able to imagine this clearly, the emotions that are experienced with imagery will be indicative of the feelings that would be experienced in the actual situation, and from this, we can have some clues about the individual's self-image.

◎ THERAPIES USING IMAGERY

Through imagery emerges a powerful, latent ability to influence normally unconscious physiologic processes in many bodily dimensions—including the gastrointestinal, cardiovascular, respiratory, and integumentary—to raise and lower such measures as the blood pressure and white-blood-cell count. For example, many people can inhibit the swelling and redness usually associated with the injection of histamine, one of the primary agents responsible for allergic symptoms. Simply telling a person that the area will not swell or telling the person that the area is becoming cold, is not as effective as telling the person to picture an ice cube being held on the area where the histamine was injected. The visual image of an ice cube mediates the inhibition of the histamine response.

In autogenic training, an individual repeats key phrases such as, "My arms and hands are heavy and warm," and imagines the arms and hands as warm. Within several weeks of training, a clear increase in the temperature of the arms and hands usually develops. Isolated in subzero weather, individuals skilled in autogenic training have been able to keep their extremities warm, while untrained companions suffered frostbite.

Biofeedback employs imagery. In a relaxed state, a client is encouraged to visualize the hands being in a warm bowl of water, for example, or the body floating on a cloud. Then, to increase the temperature of the fingers, the person imagines such things as holding the hands in front of a warm fireplace, or, to calm the forehead muscles, he or she imagines a sense of coolness in the forehead, imagines it being gently stroked with a damp cloth, or imagines a fuzzy feeling as though a cloud were settling on the forehead. To affect the gastrointestinal system, the client might picture himself or herself on a beach relaxing and listening to the water, feeling totally calm and peaceful. The scene of relaxation corrects gastrointestinal hyperactivity and hyperacidity.

Many practitioners have found that the healing response can be facilitated through the use of imagery. An example of this is a 19-year-old girl who, for about seven months, had warts on her big toe. The warts had been treated with liquid nitrogen and other techniques, but they always returned. In working with her, I brought her to a deep state of relaxation and suggested that she imagine she was traveling in a submarine and going down inside of her body. Then she visualized the warts from underneath. She saw roots coming down as if she were standing underneath the ground looking at the roots of a tree. She imagined that she had a blowtorch and that she burned all of the roots. About three or four days after this session, the warts began to turn a very dark color, and, within a week, they became completely black and dropped off, revealing normal skin underneath.

This imagery process of going within the body and visualizing it healing has been widely used in many other cultures, and it is now gaining credence here as a healing approach. It can be used for headaches, sore throats, skin rashes, gastrointestinal upsets, and other problems. Fundamentally, the imagery process involves going inside, visualizing the area of the body that needs to be healed, and picturing its healing. This may be done symbolically, for instance, by visualizing a backache as an eagle claw digging into the muscles of the back and then removing the claw with a pair of pliers. Or the imagery may be realistic, where the person actually visualizes white cells attacking and detroying invading bacteria.

One of the best-known applications of this technique is the work of Dr. Carl Simonton, a radiologist who works with cancer clients. Dr. Simonton teaches clients to enter a relaxed state and to imagine that they are traveling down inside their bodies. Here they visualize their tumor as a black rat eating the cells of their body, which resembles hamburger meat or a black cloud. Clients then imagine their own white cells attacking the cancer cells. They imagine it realistically, or they may imagine that the white cells are like many rat traps catching the rats. If a client is receiving radiation at this time, he or she might imagine that the radiation is like little poison darts shooting and weakening the rats. Other clients visualize the battle of their body against the cancer like the white knights fighting the black knights. They visualize the white knights, their own healing forces, winning. In Dr. Simonton's experience, people feel more positive about themselves and have more positive expectation of therapy. Statistics indicate that those people who use this process may actually have a longer survival period. Dr. Simonton has also described remarkable remissions in cases that ordinarily would not have been expected to remit.

Whether this kind of imagery actually improves recovery by specific stimulation of the antibody or phagocytic system; whether the process generally increases the state of well-being and thereby improves the chances of survival; and whether there is an actual, demonstrable improvement in lifespan are not proven. There is, nevertheless, an undeniable subjective change in clients working with this imagery process. Clients feel that they are no longer helpless, that they are doing something to help their body survive. They begin to picture themselves as being healthy and well. Their mood lifts, their appetite improves, and they have fewer side effects from medication or surgery. Interviews with people who have used relaxation and imagery techniques indicate that there is an improvement in the quality of life. People no longer focus continually on the day when they will live no more but instead focus more on each daily experience. Focusing positively on the future fosters the ability to let go of tensions about the future, thereby extracting more life and interest out of each moment. People do not retreat from their lives; rather, they begin to do things they've always wanted to do. Similar results have been obtained in working with people who have other serious diseases, such as degenerative vertebral disc disease, myositis, and multiple sclerosis.

The placebo effect can also depend a great deal upon the use of imagery, as seen in a particular case from my practice of medicine. I was asked by a client for sleeping pills to use on an upcoming trip. She had been able to learn to sleep by relaxing herself from head to toe when at home, but because she had always had difficulty falling asleep while traveling, she was quite apprehensive. Rather than give her a sleeping pill, I presented an antihistamine tablet, a "cold pill," which would have almost no effect on insomnia. I explained clearly to the client that this was a very strong pill, but because she had learned relaxation so well, she probably would not need all of it. I cut the pill in half. Then I described vividly how, upon awakening after taking only half of this pill, she would feel drowsy and groggy, and I cut the half pill in half again. I told her to take just this one quarter pill and described in detail how she would feel sleepy and groggy immediately but that she would awaken in the morning with almost no drug hangover. Upon returning from her trip, the client said she had used this one quarter of a pill for two nights and had slept deeply and that she had a small amount of "drug hangover." From this point on, she dispensed with the pill and used only the relaxation techniques with excellent results. By describing the best possible response to treatment, the person's spirits are lifted and expectations are improved. Response to treatment is more positive.

In psychotherapy, an individual may have an insight such as, "I really don't have to spend so much of my energy taking care of other people. I can take care of myself and other people will benefit from that!" This insight can be integrated into the person's life by having him or her imagine situations where the person would ordinarily overcommit to social gatherings and spend all his or her time providing for others. As the person visualizes these scenes, he or she imagines telling people to take more responsibility and to share in the duties involved. As a result, there is often a marked improvement in mood, a diminution of physical symptoms, and an increased social ability to communicate needs more clearly.

The person using age regression in psychotherapy imagines drifting back through time in a time machine or on a magic carpet. The person passes through many situations of the past in which maladaptive emotions, symptoms, or responses were noted. By actually picturing himself or herself in these situations and experiencing associated feelings, the person gains new insight. Following this, the person may review the situation, rewrite the script, and imagine himself or herself handling each situation in a new fashion.

Perhaps one of the most dramatic uses of age regression is when the person goes back to the critical event where he or she first began dealing with things in a certain way. A client who was completely unable to stay alone, and thus was extremely dependent on other people, regressed to an experience of being left at school the first day of kindergarten. He was the only person in the class who cried, and everyone laughed and made fun of him. As he went through this memory, many of the feelings returned, and he cried again. The experience was cathartic. The emotional insight gained was of great importance; following this session, he no longer experienced strong anxieties when parting from people.

In crisis intervention and anxiety control, acutely disturbed persons can be helped by sitting and listening carefully while a series of relaxation instructions are given. Relaxation instructions are in themselves imagery, for example, "Feel your arms and legs growing heavy; feel as though you are floating up into the air; imagine that all the tension in your body is like a black fluid and is draining out through the tips of your toes." Taking the person to a very relaxed scene in the past, or having the person picture that the ordeal is over and several weeks have passed, can result in a calm state. Upon cessation of the imagery, the individual generally feels more confident, more in touch with positive possibilities, and more functional. The imagery can be done in five to twenty minutes and might be employed when a person is acutely disturbed by being suddenly fired, for instance, or when a relationship breaks up or a major school or career failure takes place.

Imagery is also effective in helping people eliminate unwanted and maladaptive habit patterns, as in the case of an overweight client. She described her eating habits to me, and it was clear that the time she most often ate excessively was immediately after coming home from teaching school each day. She came into the house and walked straight to the refrigerator. After entering relaxation, I asked her to visualize herself driving home from work thinking about playing tennis. I had her imagine coming in the door, setting her things down, and going directly through her kitchen into the bedroom where she put on her tennis outfit. She imagined herself walking past the refrigerator, seeing it as she passed by, and feeling a surge of joy as she went straight out to play tennis. By linking the positive feelings of playing tennis with the imagery of walking past the refrigerator in order to play, a new behavior pattern became available. She did this each day upon returning from work and quickly lost her extra weight.

Another area of habit change addressed by imagery is smoking problems. Dr. Herbert Mann[3] treats people to help them cut down or stop smoking. Bringing them first to a deeply relaxed state, he asks them to imagine a burning pile of dried, decaying vegetable matter. He then has people imagine sticking their heads in the irritating, acrid cloud of smoke arising from these leaves. People find this a most unpleasant image. He paints a clear picture of this rotten vegetable matter wrapped in clean, white pieces of paper, thus associating the image of the burning pile of leaves with smoking cigarettes. Following this imagery, people find cigarettes to be distasteful, and they are able to diminish their smoking or to stop it completely. Usually, people also experience a change in confidence and ability to accomplish things, since they feel success in breaking a bad habit.

A person can use imagery in relaxation for maintaining balance in a stressful lifestyle. The client learns to relax periodically and to scan the body, looking for tense or uncomfortable areas. He or she then uses imagery to envision these places calming down. A person can use relaxation and imagery before an important interview or other stressful event. The desired outcome of interviews, business meetings, relationships, and other endeavors can be creatively visualized. Using guided imagery along with enjoyable music can enhance a person's ability to imagine positive outcomes and thus maintain a healthy balance in the system.

Imagery is also used as an adjunct to other therapies. In the Alexander technique, for instance, the person imagines his or her head floating up like a balloon as he or she walks. In certain of the Feldenkrais exercises, the individual imagines being a baby and lying on his or her back and moving the legs as a baby does.[4] In seeing a breathing therapist, an individual might be asked to focus on breathing and to imagine that the chest is lifting and falling all by itself. He or she may be asked to breathe in certain ways, for example, to imagine the breath coming in one nostril and going out the other. The approach thus uses both visual and kinesthetic imagery. In psychic approaches to healing, auras, symbols, and energy patterns are often visualized by the healer and used in diagnosis and treatment. In different forms of meditation, auditory imagery is used. Certain sounds, or a mantra, are made and repeated in the mind as though the sounds are being played on a phonograph or tape recorder. And, in energy approaches to health, the energy moving through the body may be imagined as a liquid, color, or sound.

◎ THERAPEUTIC OUTCOME

Change usually occurs simultaneously in several dimensions of the person when imagery is employed. A person who had stage fright, for example, would have been accustomed to experiencing gastric hydromotility, tension of the neck muscles, headache, and perhaps even diarrhea as a result of the fear. Along with the elimination of stage fright, we would expect to see a diminution or perhaps complete disappearance of the associated physical symptoms. A person who uses imagery to warm his or her hands to diminish the severity and incidence of migraine headaches would also have a technique of relaxing in situations in which he or she might otherwise feel anxious or tense. A person who successfully changed a maladaptive habit would feel increased self-confidence.

In imagery, the client really takes most of the responsibility for self-healing. The therapist is a guide who shows the client how to use tools that he or she already possesses. If the client learns the general techniques of relaxing and using imagery, then he or she will be capable of initiating change in the future. If the client also learns the concepts underlying relaxation and imagery techniques, he or she can initiate positive changes without needing the practitioner at all.

A limitation to the use of imagery and relaxation approaches is that all people do not respond to the same degree; there is a bell curve of responsiveness. This range of responsiveness is roughly similar to the index of suggestibility or hypnotizability.[5] Perhaps 30 percent of the people will relate very easily to these approaches. Another 40 percent will respond quite well if they are given an opportunity to practice and learn relaxation and imagery. Approximately 15 to 20 percent will find it difficult to use these techniques, although an individual who initially has difficulty using the techniques may ultimately be the person who gets the most benefit. This is true of highly intellectual people and linear thinkers. Finally, it has been found by a number of investigators that 5 to 10 percent of the population simply will not sit still to learn this particular technique.

For the practitioner who is beginning to use imagery techniques, it is better to work primarily with people in the first two groups. The ability to use this technique effectively is based upon positive experiences of it. Once a practitioner has experienced a person really making positive changes in his or her lifestyle and healing mental, physical, and emotional imbalances, then the practitioner's own belief and conviction will be greater.

Lay practitioners of imagery therapy often overstate its effectiveness. A client may become foolishly convinced that a technique can substitute for a healthy lifestyle. A person might think that imagining himself or herself running five miles a day or eating the right foods will, in some magical way, replace actually doing this. Similarly, from a psychiatric point of view, an individual who needs to develop improved family relations and communication skills would be distracted by creating imagery of himself or herself living alone and not needing to communicate with others.

Additionally, an imagery practitioner must recognize when imagery is inappropriate, such as when, for example, a client has an organic disease that requires immediate medical attention. An individual who complains of shakiness in performing a task might be thought to have stage fright or anxiety, whereas this person could have a spinal cord or mid-brain tumor. Just as the psychiatrist needs to be able to diagnose non-psychiatric causes for symptoms that appear in the psychological sphere so, too, the practitioner of imagery and relaxation must be capable of making a medical diagnosis or at least be cognizant of when to refer an individual for a medical work-up.

REFERENCES ───────────────────────────────────────

1. Maxwell Maltz, *Psychocybernetics*. (Englewood Cliffs, NJ: Prentice-Hall, Inc., 1960).

2. Carl Simonton, Stephanie Mathews-Simonton, and Jim Creighton, *Getting Well Again: A Step-By-Step Self-Help Guide To Overcoming Cancer for Patients and Their Families* (Los Angeles: J.P. Tarcher, 1978).

3. Herbert Mann, Personal communication.

4. Wilfred Barlow, *The Alexander Technique* (New York: Alfred A. Knopf, 1976).

5. Stanford Scale of Hypnotic Susceptibility. Stanford University.

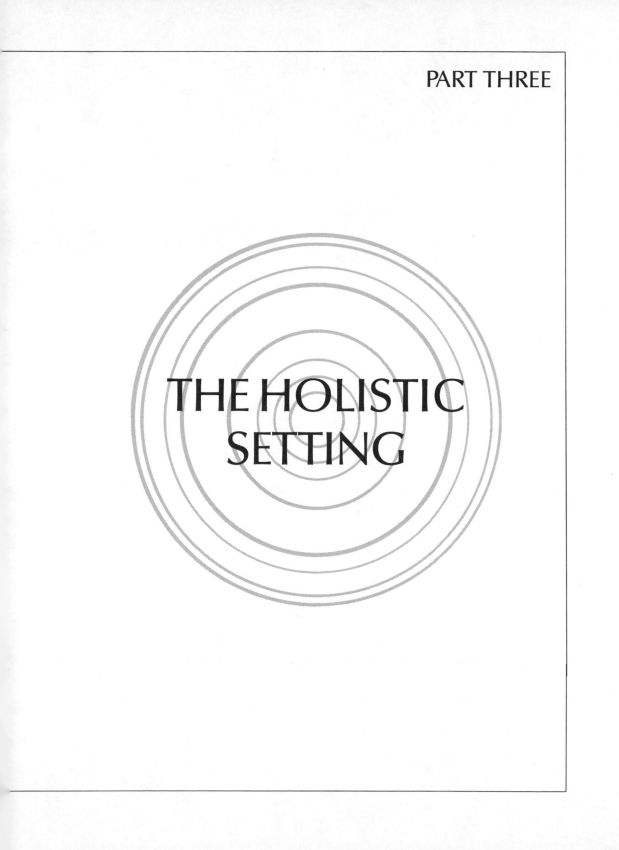

PART THREE

THE HOLISTIC
SETTING

13

THE HEALING RELATIONSHIP

HECTOR GOA, M.D.

Holism confronts science with its ignorance by dealing with the human being as a whole instead of dissecting him. Holism transports us to that frontier between man and the universe where man is a part who somehow does not know how to participate. At man's ordinary level of consciousness, he does not experience himself as a whole, a preliminary step to opening his eyes to a level of real participation and real relationship.

Holism must base its approach on the development of human consciousness, starting with the therapist. Otherwise we would just be theorizing about a sophisticated, intellectual issue. We would keep the entire pursuit at a superficial and external level, avoiding disquieting insights we have when our life does not flow smoothly.

The only possibility for being holistic is in the present moment, now, in the encounter between healer and client. The present is so precise that it can guide in discriminating between reality and fantasy, between relationship and alienation. In this encounter in the present, we find that relationships to others are either words or reactions unless we make the contact through our self. Only our whole life can relate to another life. Attempts to relate to others without this detour through the rest of our self only bring about the sentimentality or violence of our insensitive delirium and sluggish psyche.

We must leap into the unknown in order to be sincere. Do we have the courage to abandon the comfort of our identity and the pleasure of what is familiar? Can we bear the open question of life, the mystery of being aware that we really don't know and that we are not worthy of the role we are entrusted with? Are we able to trust this movement as therapeutic, even though it apparently takes us away from our skills?

We must equate health with being in constant movement and value this move toward inner silence, toward conscious sensitivity. We must try it simultaneously in front of the suffering person. Without the guidance of this active awareness of our whole body, our thought is alienated. This alienation then flows out of the healer and reinforces the client's imbalance.

It is really of balance that we are speaking when we refer to health—a balance that will allow the relaxation necessary for inner communication and sincerity. In our ordinary state of imbalance, we have no choice but to lie constantly. We don't have enough information when we manifest; we don't even have the chance to realize that there are contradictions in the information that we have already gathered.

The silent move inward, towards the unknown rest of our self, can be the thread toward continuity and real existence; like the centripetal force holding a planet in orbit and keeping it from flying off into outer space.

Holistic health must address the deepest and highest questions of man first and must start from the beginning. Only then can we remain balanced and oriented in front of the specific question brought to us. Only then can we respond without stopping movement, without disrespecting the person.

We can be genuine in our holism by including this balancing movement in our awareness, by including ourselves as part of the treatment, by moving towards direct knowledge of the other person as we make contact with higher and more intelligent parts of our presence.

Movement is the challenge. As we equilibrate between these two opposing movements, we are, at the same time, opened as a channel for higher healing forces. Even stopping to make a comment about our experience upsets the balance, closing this gate. When we lose our balance, we become unworthy of being a healer.

When we start at the beginning, putting the whole of our weight on the first step, we go further into the healing relationship. We are not just theoretical and therefore illusory. We can respond to requests for help by moving a step deeper, by opening a loving challenge, an invitation to live, to move.

The discrimination necessary to stay on this fine line of behavior can only come from the sensitivity and freedom of a balanced state. Only if we are freer than another can we help him or her. There can be no cheating. We have to pay for that freedom. Only our payment authorizes us to be an authority to another person. No social convention can replace the precise event when two human beings meet in a therapeutic circumstance.

If psychopathology and alienation could be seen as being degrees of restriction in freedom, then we can see that a hierarchy of interpersonal freedom has to be an ingredient in any authentic therapeutic relationship. A healer can never promote dependency and slavery on the part of the client but instead must promote individuation and understanding if he or she wants to be faithful to himself or herself. The therapist wants hungry men to become fishermen, not to open up a fishmarket. The therapist really has the same feeling for them that he or she has developed for himself or herself. The therapist is not alone anymore.

So the main focus shifts from hunger to the fact that a potential in the person needs to be realized. Maybe the hunger should not get response, or at least should not be totally satisfied. This hunger can be really helpful if it leads in the opposite direction, in the direction of real satisfaction, toward food that will complete the human being and help him or her feel at home.

A new, finer discrimination from our own search can give us the necessary resolution to be precise enough. This balanced attitude that we equate with health in relationships permits an openness to life and a responsiveness to life's constantly changing movements that happens when a person has mastered the fear of life. As long as we are afraid of living, we are tense and closed to the constant movement of our inner and outer lives, and we are unable to bridge the two.

Underneath, we are usually afraid of living simply because we do not know life's meaning or our meaning. We are afraid of dying. When we trust enough to open up a little, we immediately perceive the mystery in life. We experience the fear of silence and its freedom. So we shut the door by falling back into our familiar roles and our reassuring conversations until we are quiet enough to again be receptive to the present with its constantly new impressions.

Our roles and our ordinary relationships are devices to keep us separate from the flow of life, from the awareness of our ignorance, and from the information that can alleviate our fear of solitude. These relationships result from our unconscious service to powerful forces such as sex and conditioning. It means there is something essentially wrong with the ground of our relationships. In reality, we lack a relationship.

This is our situation. We are in the grip of fear, most of which is unconscious. It is the result of our attachment to the familiar, no matter how miserable it may be, which dresses us in comfortable clothes and protects us from the constant challenge of life and the responsibility of sincerely manifesting as a whole. So, we react only in our habitual ways.

Some people are motivated to free themselves from this slavery; some are not. Motivated people persist enough to make significant progress, while the rest of us remain. Even when we remain where we are, we can have a more or less gratifying relational life. Once we realize our inadequacy, motivation returns us to ourselves, in silent movement.

This process of returning to our self brings with it the possibility of witnessing our inadequacy and also our refusal to serve what is higher in our self. This calls for suffering and acceptance, the only way to go if we really want to rise above the level of judgments and division. This acceptance is the key to a right attitude toward another person—a holistic attitude.

This is why a holistic approach without an active inner work of the therapist is an illusion. Such an approach also creates a subjective hierarchy in which the healer damages himself or herself by feeding the ego satisfaction of being a guru. Inner activity and obedience are difficult: they leave no room for ego trips. We cannot go very far in the search for our self without help from others who began before us— others who are living knowledge.

A line needs to be drawn between psychopathology and inner development. The healer's responsibility is to create the conditions for distilling the client's question into a guide for the client's own search. To go beyond this point is antitherapeutic. The person should be able to go back to his or her life with relevant answers and a value for questioning himself or herself as a process. What follows after that is not the responsibility of the therapist. If the conditions are right, the client's question, like a seed, will germinate. If not, at least we have not interfered with the questioning process.

14

IDEALS FOR THE HOLISTIC HEALTH CENTER

JACK DOWNING, M.D.

Regarding free circulation as the condition of health—it is very clear that strong circulation brings health and new possibilities to all parts of an organism. Where there is constriction, disease strikes. I think that is true on all scales. It is obviously so in the body.

Rodney Collin

A Protestant minister was part-time chaplain to the San Mateo Juvenile Detention Home. Walking along the cold, anonymous concrete corridor of the girls' wing, he came upon a nine-year-old child crying bitterly. He picked her up as he would his own child and comforted her. For this, he was severely reprimanded, nearly fired, and had to settle for a note of censure being placed on his record. He kept his position only because of his previous outstanding record and his many official friends.

A shy young man began to show schizophrenic symptoms and was hospitalized. Young women nurse trainees rotated monthly through his ward as part of their training program. They would each be assigned one patient to "relate to" during that month and would spend several hours a day three days a week with him or her. A lovely, warm, young woman took a particular interest in this young man, who became much better. At the end of the month, she left and was not seen again. A week later he hanged himself.

An aging military veteran in eastern Kansas suffered an infection of the skull bones that ate away half his skull, leaving the brain exposed. After healing, he had to wear a football helmet to avoid injury. His wife refused to have sex with him, so he regularly made his way to a whorehouse in Kansas City. In retaliation, she swore out an allegation that he was mentally ill, citing the skull condition and the whorehouse visits as proof. The judge committed him to the Topeka Veteran's Hospital, where he was kept on a locked ward. The fact that he, a 60-year-old, frequently masturbated was entered in the hospital record as evidence of mental illness. The wife enjoyed his disabled veteran's pension undisturbed.

My wife, when a strapping healthy woman in her twenties, suffered a kidney infection. Wanting the best, I sent her to Stanford Hospital. When she arrived, she was told to remove her clothes and put on a skimpy hospital gown. A urinary catheter was placed in her bladder and fastened down her leg with adhesive, then she was directed to the X-ray three floors away. The elevator was crowded with fully-clothed people. She rode three floors, clutching her gaping gown, in pain from

251

the catheter, and embarrassed by the visible catheter tube showing below her gown.

An outstanding psychiatrist and captain in the United States Public Health Service decided to retire from government service. A complete physical examination was required, and he was directed to enter Bethesda Naval Hospital for the physical. He arrived, expecting a chance to play golf on the hospital course and loaf in the officers' club. The charge nurse admitted him to the ward, demanded his clothing in exchange for a hospital gown, and confined him to strict bed rest. His protests that he was completely healthy were disregarded. His rank was irrelevant. He was a patient; that's all.

We are social animals, and coming together in groups is inherent in our basic psychobiological nature. For mankind, nature is no longer our primary environment. We have overcome nature with our houses, buildings, and so forth, so that our primary environment is now society. Within society, people set up organizations or institutions to benefit people. These institutions can offer efficiency of purpose by gathering together people with related skills and needs. Any institution depends on people for its purpose and for its membership. Some people form the staff of these organizations, while others receive service intermittently from the organization. However, institutions also have a life independent of individuals. From government to marriage, institutions develop rules and habits over time that often outlast generations of people.

We have extended organizations beyond the small, flexible group (usually about a dozen people) where people can have person-to-person relations. We have organized ourselves into enormous institutions in which rules have to be set up; in which, for smooth operation, there have to be some fixed guides to behavior. We need conventions.

Over time, rules originally established to ensure that the institution runs smoothly often become inflexible. Rules may become so rigid that they no longer serve people; in fact, they oppose what the institution is supposed to be about in the first place. By maintaining such inflexible rules, institutions prevent people from getting what they truly need and prevent some people, as in the case of the minister, from *giving* others what they need. What the child in that situation needed was simple, affectionate comforting, but there were strict rules that no personnel could touch any of the inmates.

Health care institutions are, unfortunately, not exempt from these peculiarities of institutions. Consider the image that a hospital typically operates on a factory model. The out-of-repair patient enters the institution on an insurance-fueled conveyor belt to be processed, tagged, injected, and sanitized; shunted here for laboratory, there for X-rays, elsewhere for radioactivity or sonar. He or she may be tranquilized or stimulated, amputated or chordated; reamed, cleaned, shriven and shorn; carted, transported, wheeled and credit checked; perfused, transfused, confused, and subterfused; until, God and pathology willing, the once-again fully functioning patient is carefully wheeled out of the hospital and permitted to touch foot to earth only outside the insurance-set limits of the hospital. Here, the ward orderly returns the patient to his or her own custody and says, "Now watch your step, and rest up at home." Presumably, the patient/product is complete, in full repair.

Institutions operating with rigidity reduce the humanity of both the staff and the clients by their institutional rules. The cases cited show what happens in a variety of situations when people enter institutions and are objectified by institutional rules and protocol, rather than being treated as individual human beings with unique needs. Often, the way we manage to be human beings within institutions is to ignore or pervert the institutional rules. A good example of this occurs in the book *One Flew Over the Cuckoo's Nest*. But perverting or ignoring the rules isn't the solution to the problem. It should be kept in mind that institutions don't intentionally set out to dehumanize people, but the structure of many of them has built-in qualities that effectively do dehumanize. How, then, do we shape the institution so that it both maintains itself and provides what people need as human beings? Can a smoothly running health center not sicken its consumers, and can it even be health enhancing?

In recent years, many holistic health centers have been created throughout California and in other locations in the U.S. These centers, too, are institutions. Even though holistic health centers are founded upon a philosophy and approach that is different from principles held in current traditional health institutions, they, too, must deal with the peculiarities inherent in the general nature of institutions. Holistic health centers have rules and guides to behavior that staff and clients are expected to follow, and, as centers grow in size and expand in their functions, those rules may begin to calcify. It is tempting to think that holistic health centers will automatically be different because the approach is *holistic*.

Ideally, the holistic health center sets out to tend to all facets of each client and to promote well-rounded, positive health. The crucial part of treatment that makes the holistic approach holistic is the tying together or making sense of all the facets of the client being treated. If the holistic health center ends up operating on the traditional institutional or factory model, then by the definition of holism itself, the center would not be holistic because it couldn't make those essential connections. It would merely be another health care institution, one with a number of alternative types of therapies available but equally capable of dehumanizing clients.

Holistic health centers do have the potential to change the way health care institutions evolve and operate, and they have the potential to be health enhancing for their clients. Among the several holistic health principles that can be used to facilitate this goal, two interrelated principles especially apply. One is that each part of the health organization has a distinct integrity and, simultaneously, a functional identity with the whole, so the parts will reflect the nature of the whole. The other is that the client is an integral part of the center and, as such, must take responsibility for himself or herself.

◎ "HOLISM" IN THE HEALTH CENTER

Systems usually operate as wholes. Various levels or parts of a system have similar qualities, much as each portion of a hologram can reproduce the whole or as each cell has enough DNA to recreate the entire organism. Similarly, the holistic health center can be considered a system, with members of its staff and treatment modalities as parts of the system. The holistic model assumes that the health of the client, practitioner, and team or center are interrelated. The center is composed of medical knowledge, and the client, practitioner, and health care team function together as one social system. If all the component parts are operating with integrity, then the health care system itself has integrity and operates at a higher, more effective level. Unfortunately, even if the component parts of the health care system don't operate with integrity, the system may still limp along for some time because it is characteristic of systems that they will continue almost regardless of what happens to people in the system. But then the quality is at stake.

Ernest Lowe elaborates the notion of integrity of system components in his listing of four basic aspects of medical wholeness.[1]

1. *The integrity of medical knowledge and the means of achieving health and wholeness*. This knowledge is global, though particular medical systems may be different.
2. *The integrity of the client*. The person is a unity of mind, body, emotion, and spirit, endowed with an innate capability of self-healing when he or she receives the necessary support and guidance.

3. *The integrity of the health practitioner*. Any improvement in the practitioner's own state of health inevitably affects his or her ability to guide others toward health.
4. *The integrity of the health care team*. A group of people working with openness, unity, and recognition of each other's human needs and gifts provides optimum conditions for health care.

The Integrity of Medical Knowledge

Health care institutions operate with an assumption of soundness of the medical knowledge and techniques used. In most cases, people are doing the best they know, and the assumption of soundness is valid. Whether the approach is modern Western, primitive, Oriental, or holistic, the fundamental goal is always health and wholeness; medical knowledge and practices are means to achieving this goal. If the medical knowledge of the health care center is the best available at any point in time because it is continually updated, then an ideal high level of integrity is maintained.

By and large, Western medicine is oriented toward symptom, cause, and treatment or cure. Trained in disease and pathology, practitioners seek to make their patients at ease and free of distress. Pharmaceutical advertising and drug literature in medical journals emphasize this simple symptom-relief care. The attractive seeming simplicity of this approach results in the high prescription rates of mind-altering drugs and widespread use of antibiotics. All over the world, where such drugs are freely available without prescription, their wide use attests to the popular appeal of this approach. The approach can sometimes relieve pain or distress sufficiently to allow a deeper look into the problem, but too often, both practitioner and patient stop treatment once the symptoms are relieved. Yet the symptom-relief approach continues because it is standard in the traditional health care model.

In the actual medical situation, what is practiced is what meets medically accepted standards. In other words, practitioners usually go ahead and do what they've always done; human knowledge is the residue of human experience gained over a long period of time. Today, we would scoff at the idea that bleeding is necessary for health, but there was a period of several hundred years in which bleeding was thought to be the only treatment for almost anything. Many people undoubtedly died of blood loss. What is interesting is that the practice was not done away with by practitioners. It was abolished by, essentially, a consumer revolt. So practitioners tend to be the guardians of the established standards and practices. If a doctor uses something too unorthodox, he or she is in danger of being censured. If the doctor does what is expected, then he or she cannot be criticized if the results do not turn out well. Medical traditions are slow to change.

What this means is that not all medical practice is valid: much of it is practice that is accepted because it is hallowed by previous tradition, not because it is the most effective practice currently available. Characteristic of all institutions and of human knowledge is the fact that something done before carries weight and validity, apart from any examination of its results. To this extent, medical knowledge and practice lose integrity, and the goals of health and wholeness cannot be fully reached.

Practices that are entirely new to the West, like applied kinesiology and acupuncture, don't fit into this pattern and are not viewed as integral to medical practice. As new ideas, they can be tried and evaluated for usefulness. Usually, such *avante garde* practices have to be tried in non-traditional settings, such as holistic health centers, or in private practices. New practices correct inertia and return us to the integrity of positive health through the best method available.

The basic objectives of positive health have been known in other cultures which, lacking specific treatment methods, have had to depend on prevention rather than cure. Let us take one traditional modality, massage, as an example. Using hands on the body is age-old. Most cultures have some form of health-enhancing, disease-removing process that involves touch with varying degrees of pressure. In European and Russian medicine, this is formalized in hydrotherapy, balncotherapy, and massage therapy and is centered principally at the great spas. In the United States, however, changes in medical education after the turn of the century set medical practice toward the scientific, biochemical, surgical, and laboratory model: treatment rather than prevention and elimination of disease rather than facilitation of health became the goals.

Manipulation and massage were left to physiotherapists and rehabilitation specialists, who sought to be as aloof and "scientific" as their more prestigious medical brethren. With neglect of preventive techniques, the system of health-oriented "watering places" or spas withered and died. Instead of baths and massage, "scientific" doctors followed the medical trends. First bromides, later barbiturates, then Librium and Valium, were prescribed. Manipulation and massage as health-promoting and healing processes were left almost entirely to osteopaths, chiropractors, and non-medical healers.

The growth of holistic health knowledge and practices is, thus, an attempt to return to older goals of positive health and wholeness.

But since the knowledge of holistic health has only recently re-entered scientific medical practice, the level of integrity in holistic medicine needs to be high to maintain credibility and effectiveness.

The Integrity of the Client

The person is a unity of mind, body, emotion, and spirit endowed with an innate capability of healing himself or herself when he or she has the motivation and receives the necessary support and guidance. The client always heals himself or herself. Whatever the method used—miracle drugs, heart transplants, person-machine couplings, faith healing, etc.—ultimately, the client always heals himself or herself. The reportedly favorable effects of visualization techniques and other forms of meditation on persons with cancer and other chronic diseases may be considered evidence of innate self-healing ability. The skillful health practitioner generates those conditions that favor recovery from illness and self-healing for the client, but the practitioner cannot actually *heal* the client. Client motivation, though, is essential to self-healing. The goal of practitioners is, then, to encourage motivation and provide the necessary support and guidance.

Aside from treatment, most chronic or complex illnesses require changes in lifestyle or in those habits that perpetuate the illness conditions. A person's existing patterns, particularly biological patterns of eating, ingestion, activity, etc., are difficult to change. Most people see a doctor because they don't feel well or they are scared, not necessarily because they know they need to change something and are looking for guidance in doing this. Usually, if the doctor simply makes them feel better, most people are satisfied, even though it may not solve the real problem. There are exceptions, like arthritis or cancer, where the person feels bad for a long period of time and is therefore willing to do anything, including change. The client who expends sincere effort in growing beyond his or her illness into a higher level of well-being and is willing to take charge of his or her health is acting with personal integrity.

In the Oriental approach to medicine, practitioners assume the integrity of the individual; they view the client as though he or she is in an unimpaired condition. Symptoms are seen as clues to understanding the imbalance, not as indications that the client is unsound. When the client is viewed by the practitioner as being pathological in some way, the client's true integrity can't be seen or realized. The same is true when the client sees himself or herself in terms of the problem, even becomes the problem, rather than seeing himself or herself as a whole person who is out of balance.

The Integrity of the Health Practitioner

Any improvement in the practitioner's state of health inevitably enhances his or her ability to guide others toward health. Health care requires energy—energy which is available for use in the service of others. The practitioner who is in better health will likely be able to see all aspects of the client more clearly and, thus, be more effective as a doctor. For the physician, adequate health practice, expressing and integrating body, mind, heart, and spirit, is prerequisite to giving adequate care and guidance to others.

Regrettably, in medicine there exists a tradition of excessive service that exhausts the capacity of the health practitioner beyond the point of being able to maintain adequate health himself or herself. Many hospitals and outpatient clinics are set up to be "highly efficient" operations, where time spent with each client is reduced so that doctors can see 40 to 50 clients per day.

In this system, the practitioner is likely to be exhausted and, further, has no time to take a holistic approach. He or she is pressured to practice medicine on a simplistic basis: a person has certain lab signs; if their cholesterol is up, the doctor puts them on a low cholesterol diet or gives them anti-cholesterol medication. If a person has hemorrhoids, the practitioner gives them hemorrhoidal ointment or has a surgeon cut the hemorrhoids out. There is no time available for the practitioner to find out why the person has hemorrhoids, what the stresses are in this person's life that have produced hemorrhoids, and what can be done about the stress. In this kind of operation, both practitioner and client lose integrity.

The holistic center expects the entire staff to be healthy rather than wealthy and overworked, to seek self-knowledge as well as technical proficiency, and to consciously provide a model for clients. The practitioner who is in excellent health will be a more credible model of health, while the one who is obviously not taking care of his or her own health will be unconvincing. Specifically, those practices such as smoking, overeating, or failing to exercise, which the center's educational program presents as harmful to clients, are equally dangerous to the practitioner. The center must support the practitioner as well as the client in identifying and using systems and disciplines that are concordant with each person's traditions and values for seeking positive health. The health center supports equally the welfare of the practitioner and of the client. Both are joined in similar goals, in asserting the privilege and responsibility of vital and vigorous involvement in the world. The health practitioner is privileged to exemplify in himself or herself a maximal way of life.

The Integrity of the Health Care Team

Teamwork in medical care seems to be taking precedence over the individual or "solo" practitioner approach, particularly in the holistic health setting. A group of people working with unity, openness, and recognition of each other's human needs and gifts provides one of the best conditions for health care because the client may be seen by several specialists tending all facets of the client. To be effective, team members must work together as a real unit. True teamwork is not learned by specialized study or on-the-job training that focuses on specific skills appropriate only to the task at hand. Teamwork skills that will reinforce the client's motivation to become more healthy are acquired by learning ego-less self-discipline that enables the health practitioner to become relatively free of immature resentments over imagined slights or underlying needs to dominate others. This leaves the practitioner free to work in full cooperation with other team members, thus ensuring the integrity of the team as a functional unit.

For most of us, our ability to work in teams is an expression of our life experience in a hierarchical society. We usually experience personal responsibility in terms of rights and obligations to an authority figure called parent, teacher, sergeant, or boss. Strong punishment-reward, negative-positive, frustration-appreciation tensions are created that, in turn, condition our successive work group relations. We tend to evade or sabotage unpleasant experiences involving self-discipline and to displace frustration downward to lower levels. This occurs internally, in relation to our own sense of responsibility, and externally in relation to social and work relationships. As a health practitioner, I can, for example, sabotage my own mature resolve to stop smoking by acting like an irresponsible child; if I am angry with my job, I can similarly sabotage the health team's goal by covertly encouraging clients to continue with smoking or other deleterious habits.

At the interpersonal, team level, the probability of both expressed and covert conflict is high. Personality friction drains the enthusiasm of a health care team just as friction slows a moving object. The result of conflict, poor communication, and/or misunderstanding is a net loss of energy and a loss of integrity for the health care team. Both the client and the center are the poorer for such malfunctioning. We have all experienced organizations that function splendidly with high spirit and good communication and others that are wretched places to be. The latter give grudging service to their clients.

Though it is difficult to eliminate the hierarchical structure from nstitutional setting, still the typical dehumanizing aspect can be ificantly minimized if no one is exempt from responsibility for di-participation in the common effort. In a large health care facility, ...istance, personnel can rotate a certain portion of their responsibilities on a monthly lottery basis. Kitchen and janitorial crews, practitioners, clients, and visitors alike can work on the grounds, in the kitchen, and at the reception desk. Tasks at many levels can be shared. These efforts minimize hierarchical forms and change vertical communication to lateral communication.

Dealing with people who are in pain, worried, and frustrated puts a load on members of the health care team. The center can provide opportunity to share and dissipate this load. Daily exercise to release tension, training in identifying and releasing tension as it occurs, and light-hearted activities are all useful. A minimum of four weeks yearly of vacation time is essential for rest and recharging of basic life energy. (In Russia, mental health practitioners are allotted six weeks, as their work is considered more stressful than regular medical practice.) Further, staff members can use the same support mechanisms provided for clients in health enhancement and education activities. Staff members can also be fully involved both in operations and in planning for procedures affecting them and their client-centered activities.

Social organizations are by nature goal-oriented and are arranged according to hierarchical levels. The holistic health center is not an exception to this reality, yet it can still incorporate an open-door, open-heart policy for free communication among staff members and between staff and clients. Love, hope, and healing are not held within hierarchical tables of organization; the way must be clear for their flow, lest we tend the form of helping and kill the spirit. Cherishing the essential equality of all human beings requires openness and sharing among staff, regardless of badges of rank such as age, position, or other distinctions.

THE CENTER AS A WHOLE

A final area of integrity in holistic health care can also be considered: the integrity of the center as a whole. Once it has achieved integrity or wholeness in its medical knowledge, clientele, staff, and health care team, the holistic health center can establish itself as a viable entity that interacts with its community responsively. From an internal standpoint, the center does this by working toward time and cost efficiency. Externally, the center builds in enough flexibility to be responsive to the real-life conditions of its clients and community, and it takes an active role in promoting positive health in its community.

In a multidisciplinary, psychiatric outpatient clinic, I did a time-utilization study. Twenty-seven percent of expensive professional staff time went into conferences with each other that were not for the purpose of dissipating tension. Thirty-six percent went into records, coffee breaks, telephoning, etc. Only 37 percent went into actual contact with clients. A public, tax-supported service got away with this degree of inefficiency for many years, and other clinics still do. It is inefficient because, for the amount clients pay in total, too little time is spent with them, and too few useful services are given. Even a simple calculation of client fees in ratio to staff salaries dictates a more efficient system. Yet it is often the case, even in the holistic model, that health centers are not time and cost effective.

In conventional clinics, a substantial portion of revenue comes from laboratory, X-ray, pharmacy, and such. Ancillary personnel doing injections, counseling, and other conventional services generate additional revenue. Insurance companies and government agencies are conditioned to view these activities as allowable charges. So, if the clinic does enough of them rapidly enough, it profits. Unfortunately, holistic centers run into two financial blocks: they don't do nearly as many lab tests, and most of their treatment procedures don't qualify for reimbursement. Holistic medicine is concerned with the whole person—every aspect of the human being—and the program of the holistic center aims beyond illness treatment to maximum health and joyfully living up to our full potential. But we must ask ourselves, can better health be the province of the medical center? Can we afford such an ambitious objective? Where do we get the resources, and who will pay?

Even though there is substantial popular dissatisfaction with value received in conventional medicine, the general populace is slow to change to holistic treatments. Undoubtedly, part of the reason is that people must pay for all of it straight from their pockets. It is sad, but true, that potential clients go where their money goes farthest, so many clients choose conventional health care centers primarily because their health insurance or company insurance covers the costs. Unless holistic health centers get the quickening flow of these third-party payments irrigating the channels of their accounts, they'll remain poor relations compared to the rest of the medical establishment. A requirement for mutual co-responsibility between client and center is that the holistic health center be self-supporting by a combination of direct and third-party payment.

Yet, preventive medicine can actually be more cost effective than remedial treatment. The Kaiser Foundation health care system has found that unlimited outpatient treatment lowers overall cost by decreasing hospitalization. Also, the rise of community mental health centers and closing of state hospitals for therapy has at least been cost allowable. We can reasonably assume that avoiding illness is more efficient than treating symptoms. As Mother used to say, "Good food is cheaper than medicine."

Positive health intervention is not new. Assisting another person to become healthy and avoid illness is the traditional province of public health. The successes of this field of medicine are many and greatly honored. Certainly, mass vaccination was less costly than mass treatment of smallpox. However, since the obvious successes, such as pure water, disease vector control, and pasteurized milk have been accomplished, we are dealing with harder, more complex problems requiring individual motivation for habit change and self-discipline. Habits of eating, drinking, smoking, exercise, work and family relationships, and relationship to self and to ethical, social, and religious systems are all deeply involved in health promotion and illness prevention. In one area, coronary artery disease, a rise in public consciousness with resulting wide improvement in diet and exercise does seem to correlate with a lowering of the heart disease death rate in the last decade after 50 years of a rising incidence.

As part of its role in interacting with the community, the health center can modify or revise its structure to offer services to other population groups whose life situation may be tougher for the staff to appreciate and treat. For example, groceries available in a blue-collar superette grocery store, the only convenient food source in many areas, are grossly deficient in nutrients and high in fat and carbohydrates. Many people live on this diet. Much illness, direct and indirect, results from such hidden malnutrition. The center can form community outreach programs to offer information on nutrition and help bring about changes in the quality of food available for the money. Instruction and related therapeutic practices in problem areas like this must not be idealized but rather tailored to clients' actual social and economic situations. By recognizing the shared responsibility for health among client, practitioner, center, and community, the holistic health center can be in an excellent position to improve client motivation and to affect positively the health of the community.

THE INDIVIDUAL AS AN INTEGRAL PART OF THE ORGANIZATION

To be treated as a human being rather than as an object, the client must take an active as well as a receptive role in health care. The holistic health center's staff can be oriented toward helping to inspire the client's individual motivation in this direction. The center must be partner, not priest, to the health-seeking person or family, combining treatment with prevention and instruction. The client must begin becoming responsible by letting go of the idea that the doctor is going to do everything for the client and that all decisions, diagnoses, and treatments are entirely up to the doctor. As the client becomes more responsible for his or her own health, he or she is usually more aware of the subtleties of symptoms and can contribute to a more accurate diagnosis. The client can help determine which treatment or therapy most suits him or her and then take responsibility for carrying out the therapy. Clients can also actively participate in the center's health-enhancing programs and can be openly receptive to new treatment modalities.

The center cannot be responsible for what the individual actually does to and for himself or herself. At some point in the relationship between center and client, both parties must recognize this fact of co-responsibility and negotiate and implement a mutual contract. In my practice, for example, I use a simple contract with my clients. It reads as follows:

> I know that my health is my own responsibility, in partnership with Dr. Downing. I agree to carry out the program outlined below. If I want to change or drop the program, I will talk with Dr. Downing before doing so.
>
> I agree that I will keep all appointments, except under serious circumstances. If I cancel, I will give 24 hours notice or be charged my regular hourly fee. My fee will be paid at each visit, with any insurance being paid to me.

The program lists details of diet, vitamins, medication, and recreational drugs that the client may be taking, their duration/evaluation, and other practitioners or modalities. I check back with clients, and if they are not complying with our contract, I say, "Alright, if not this, then what else are you able to do?" The doctor can propose; the client has to dispose. The client almost always agrees with the doctor in the office but often finds that he or she can't or won't carry out the program afterwards. A Philadelphia study done many years ago showed that only one third of the medications prescribed by doctors were actually taken. A contract is a partial solution, but in general, greater client responsibility can ensure a better working relationship between center or practitioner and client and improved health for the client.

Even the semantics of this center/client partnership can be used to advantage. For example, the health-seeking individual may be referred to as the *client* rather than the *patient*. *Patient* implies passivity and lack of volition, whereas *client* suggests activity—the seeking of services and active partnership. The more initiative and responsibility the client feels at the center, the more he or she can examine the unique details of his or her own illness and then cultivate and maintain new, healthier practices.

The stress-adaptation concept of Hans Selye is a useful tool at this point. Stress produced by an illness condition requires adaptation, and the admission of any new client to a health care center also produces stress and requires adaptation for both parties. Life stress demands adaptation if the person undergoing stress is to survive and thrive. Adaptation means that the physical body and the whole person respond to changes in environment by making adjustments to meet the changed conditions. Stress of any kind evokes an adaptation response. Stress is not, in itself, abnormal; all new experiences are essentially changes in environment and are stressful since they demand adaptation. Upon entering a health center, the client adapts to the center, and the center adapts to the client. Various outcomes are possible, particularly in the long-term client/center relationship:

1. If the adaptation is successful, client and center join, and the energy of the total system is enhanced. Both client and center grow and benefit. Both center and client succeed in making modifications and reducing stress.

2. The health center may adapt to the stress of a new client by regarding him or her as an outsider, alien, and an intruder, to be processed and ejected as soon as possible. In this instance, adaptation is not successful for either party; thus stress remains for both, and the relationship is most likely terminated.

3. The client may be accepted in a limited, dependent patient role that exaggerates the scope and authority of the health team. In contrast to the client's enforced incapacity and dependency, the health professional is then seen as a powerful individual to be highly regarded. In this case, adaptation is only partial, and stress is not sufficiently reduced to be health enhancing.

Traditional health care institutions frequently do reduce the stress of adaptation to illness for the client by giving medical requests for sick leave, prescriptions for tranquilizers, and consultations with important or effective personages. As short-term actions, these may be salutary, but as long-term methods, they can actually reduce the client's general adaptational skills, distracting him or her from careful attention to diet, movement, relaxation, or relationships—at times even producing addictions and medication allergies.

As an alternative, by guiding the mutual adaptation, the holistic health center can model a way of handling stress that the client can continue to use in life. For example, a client with allergic asthma may not have noticed that the asthma attacks come on in certain kinds of emotional situations, such as during an exam or a conference with the foreman. If the client is guided to realizing this, he or she can take steps in advance to avoid an asthmatic attack: increase the nebulizer inhaler dosage, make dietary changes, etc. Many men complain of impotence with high blood pressure medication. The health care center can agree with the man in advance to give him the necessary medication to get his blood pressure down and simultaneously develop with him a diet and exercise regime that will enable him to decrease the medication and still keep his blood pressure down. Thus, the client learns to handle stress intelligently instead of becoming symptomatic.

In summary, a comprehensive health care center serves to integrate the client into a positive health attitude, treat the symptoms as needed, and use appropriate educational and other measures to raise the client's stress adaptational and healing abilities. The practitioner and health care system can influence the client toward or away from true health. The system must allow the client some influence along with self-responsibility. The reciprocal nature of the client/system relationship must be recognized to evolve a flexible treatment system that can operate swiftly, subtly, and effectively.

REFERENCES

1. Ernest Lowe (unpublished notes, 1975).

Bajema, Carl Jay. *Natural Selection in Human Populations.* New York: John Wiley & Sons, Inc., 1971.

Ballentine, Rudolph. *Diet & Nutrition, a Holistic Approach.* Honesdale, PA: Himalayan International Institute, 1978.

Ballentine, Rudolph; Swami Rama; and Hymes, Alan. *Science of Breath, A Practical Guide.* Honesdale, PA: Himalayan International Institute, 1979.

Ballentine, Rudolph; Swami Rama; and Swami Ajaya. *Yoga and Psychotherapy.* Honesdale, PA: Himalayan International Institute, 1979.

Bandler, Richard, and Grinder, John. *The Structure of Magic, Vols. 1 and 2.* Palo Alto, CA: Science and Behavior, 1975.

Barefoot Doctor's Guide (The American Translation of the Official Chinese Paramedical Manual). Philadelphia: Running Press, 1977.

Barlow, W. *The Alexander Technique.* New York: Alfred A. Knopf, Inc., 1973.

Basmajian, J. V., ed. *Biofeedback—Principles and Practice for Clinicians.* Baltimore, MD: Williams & Wilkins Co., 1978.

Bateson, Gregory. *Steps to an Ecology of Mind.* New York: Ballantine Books, Inc., 1972.

Beau, Georges. *Chinese Medicine.* New York: Avon Publishers, 1972.

Benson, Herbert. *The Mind/Body Effect.* New York: Simon & Schuster, Inc., 1979.

————. *The Relaxation Response.* New York: William Morrow & Company, 1975.

Berkeley Holistic Health Center. *The Holistic Health Handbook.* Berkeley, CA: And-Or Press, 1978.

Bettelheim, Bruno. *The Informed Heart.* New York: Free Press of Glencoe, 1960.

Biofeedback Society of California. *Handbook and Directory,* 1976.

Birk, L., ed. *Biofeedback: Behavioral Medicine.* New York: Grune & Stratton, 1973.

Birren, Faber. *Color Psychology and Therapy.* Secaucus, NJ: University Books, 1961.

Blackie, Margery G. *The Patient, Not the Cure.* London: MacDonald & Jane's, 1976.

Bloomfield, Harold H., and Kory, Robert B. *The Holistic Way to Health and Happiness.* New York: Simon & Schuster, Inc., 1978.

Bloomfield, Harold; Cain, M.; and Jaffe, R. *TM: Discovering Inner Energy and Overcoming Stress.* New York: Delacorte Press, 1975.

BIBLIOGRAPHY

Academy of Traditional Chinese Medicine. *An Outline of Chinese Acupuncture*. Peking: Foreign Language Press, 1975.

Achterberg, J.; Simonton, O. C.; and Matthews-Simonton, S. *Stress, Psychological Factors, and Cancer*. Fort Worth, TX: New Medicine Press, 1976.

Airola, Paavo O. *Health Secrets from Europe*. New York: Arco Publishing Company, 1972.

———. *How To Get Well*. Phoenix, AZ: Health Plus Publishers, 1974.

Alexander, F. *Psychosomatic Medicine*. New York: W. W. Norton & Co., Inc 1950.

———. *The Resurrection of the Body*. New York: Delta, 1969.

Alford, Robert R. *Health Care Politics*. Chicago: University of Chica Press, 1975.

Alland, Alexander, Jr. *Adaptation in Cultural Evolution: An Approach Medical Anthropology*. New York: Columbia University Press, 1970.

Ardell, Donald. *High Level Wellness*. Emmaus, PA: Rodale Press, Inc., 19

Arms, Suzanne. *Immaculate Deception*. Boston: Houghton Mifflin, 1975

Assagioli, Roberto. *Psychosynthesis*. New York: Viking Press, 1965.

Bach, Edward. *Heal Thyself*. London: C. W. Daniel, 1978. (Originally lished in 1931.)

Blum, Henrik L. *Expanding Health Care Horizons*. Oakland, CA: Third Party Press, 1976.

Blum, R. *The Management of the Doctor-Patient Relationship*. New York: McGraw-Hill Book Co., 1960.

Boadella, David. *Wilhelm Reich: The Evolution of His Work*. London: Vision, 1974.

Bonny, H. L., and Savary, L. M. *Music and Your Mind: Listening with a New Consciousness*. New York: Harper & Row Publishers, Inc., 1973.

Boston Women's Health Book Collective. *Our Bodies, Ourselves,* 2d ed. New York: Simon & Schuster, Inc. 1976.

Boxerman, David, and Spilken, Aron. *Alpha Brain Waves, Meditation, Biofeedback, and Altered States of Consciousness*. Millbrae, CA; Celestial Arts Publishing Co., 1975.

Boyd, Doug. *Rolling Thunder*. New York: Random House, Inc., 1974.

Bresler, David E. *Electrophysiological and Behavioral Correlates of Acupuncture Therapy*. International Symposium on Pain, Seattle, Washington, 1973.

Bresler, David E., and Trubo, Richard. *Free Yourself from Pain*. New York: Simon & Schuster, Inc., 1979.

Bricklin, Mark. *Natural Healing Cookbook*. Emmaus, PA: Rodale Press, Inc., 1981.

―――. *The Practical Encyclopedia of Natural Healing*. Emmaus, PA: Rodale Press, Inc. 1976.

Brody, Howard. The Systems View of Man: Implications for Science, Medicine and Ethics. *Perspectives in Biology and Medicine,* Autumn, 1973: 71–92.

Brody, Howard, and Sobel, David. A Systems View of Health and Disease. *Ways of Health: Holistic Approaches to Ancient and Contemporary Medicine,* ed. D. Sobel, New York: Harcourt, Brace, Jovanovich, Inc., 1979.

Brooks, Charles. *Sensory Awareness*. New York: Viking Press, Inc., 1974.

Brown, B. *New Mind, New Body*. New York: Harper & Row Publishers, Inc., 1975.

Butler, Robert N. *Why Survive? Being Old in America*. New York: Harper & Row Publishers, Inc., 1975.

Campbell, Joseph. *The Masks of God: Creative Mythology*. New York: Penguin Books, Inc., 1968.

Cannon, W. B. Voodoo Death. *American Anthropologist* 44: 169.

Capra, Fritjof. *The Tao of Physics*. Boulder, CO: Shambhala Publications, Inc., 1975.

Carlson, Rick J. *The End of Medicine.* New York: Wiley-Interscience, 1975.

Carroll, David. *The Complete Book of Natural Medicines.* New York: Summit Books, 1980.

Carter, Mildred. *Hand Reflexology: Key to Perfect Health.* New York: Parker Publishing Company, 1975.

Cassell, Eric, J. *The Healer's Art.* New York: J.B. Lippincott Company, 1976.

Castaneda, Carlos. *Tales of Power.* New York: Simon & Schuster, Inc., 1974.

———. *Journey to Ixtlan.* New York; Simon & Schuster, Inc., 1973.

———. *A Separate Reality.* New York: Simon & Schuster, Inc., 1971.

———. *The Teachings of Don Juan.* New York: Ballantine Books, 1968.

Cheek, David B., and Lecron, Leslie M. *Clinical Hypnotherapy.* New York: Grune & Stratton, 1968.

Cheraskin, E., and Ringsdorf, W.M. *Predictive Medicine.* Mountain View, CA: California Pacific Press, 1973.

Cheraskin, E., Ringsdorf, W.M., Jr.; and Clark, J.W. *Diet and Disease.* New Canaan, CT: Keats Publishing, Inc., 1977.

Churchman, C. West. *Design of Inquiring Systems, Basic Concepts in Systems Analysis.* New York: Basic Books, Inc., 1972.

Clynes, Manfred. *Sentics: The Touch of the Emotions.* Garden City, NY: Anchor Press/Doubleday, Inc., 1978.

Coddington, Mary. *In Search of the Healing Energy.* New York: Warner/Destiny Books, 1978.

Comfort, Alex. *A Good Age.* Avenel, NJ: Crown Publishers, Inc., 1976.

Cooper, K.H. *Aerobics.* New York: Bantam Books, Inc., 1976.

Coulter, Harris L. *Homeopathic Medicine.* Washington, D.C.: American Foundation for Homeopathy, 1972.

Cousins, Norman. Anatomy of an Illness (As Perceived by the Patient). *New England Journal of Medicine.* 295 (26): 1458-1463.

Cox, H. *Turning East: The Promise and Peril of the New Orientalism.* New York: Simon & Schuster, Inc., 1978.

Crasilneck, Harold B., and Hall, James A. *Clinical Hypnosis: Principles and Applications.* New York: Grune & Stratton, 1975.

De Beauvoir, Simone. *The Coming of Age.* New York: Warner Publications, 1973.

———. *A Very Easy Death.* New York: Penguin Books, 1969.

Deliman, Tracy. The Integration of Acupuncture and Chinese Medicine into the Western Medical System. Unpublished Master's Thesis. San Francisco: San Francisco State University, 1978.

Dextreit, Raymond. *Our Earth, Our Cure.* Translated by Michael Abehsera. New York: Swan House, 1974.

Dick-Read, Grantly. *Childbirth Without Fear.* 2d. rev. ed. New York: Harper & Row Publishers, Inc., 1970.

Dilfer, Carol. *Your Baby, Your Body.* New York: Crown Publishers, Inc., 1977.

Dintenfass, Julius. *Chiropractic: A Modern Way to Health.* New York: Pyramid Books, 1975.

Dong, Collin H., and Banks, Jane. *New Hope for the Arthritic.* New York: Ballantine Books, Inc., 1975.

Dorland's Illustrated Medical Dictionary. Philadelphia: W. B. Saunders Co., 1974.

Downing, George. *Massage and Meditation.* New York: Random House, Inc., 1974.

———. *The Massage Book.* New York: Random House, Inc., 1973.

Downing, Jack. *Gestalt Awareness.* New York: Harper & Row Publishers, Inc., 1976.

Downing, Jack, and Marmorstein, Robert. *Dreams and Nightmares.* New York: Harper & Row Publishers, Inc., 1972.

Downing, Jack; Lamb, Richard; and Heath, Don. *Handbook of Community Mental Health.* San Francisco: Jossey-Bass Inc., Publishers, 1969.

Dreitzel, Hans Peter. *The Social Organization of Health.* New York: Macmillan Publishing Company, Inc., 1971.

Dubos, Rene. *Mirage of Health.* New York: Harper & Row Publishers, Inc., 1971.

———. *Man, Medicine and Environment.* New York: Praeger Publishers, 1968.

———. *So Human an Animal.* New York: Charles Scribner's Sons, 1968.

———. *Man Adapting.* New Haven, CT: Yale University Press, 1965.

Duke, Marc. *Acupuncture.* New York: Pyramid House, 1972.

Dunbar, F. *Psychosomatic Diagnosis.* New York: Harper & Row Publishers, Inc., 1954.

Dunbar, Flanders. *Emotions and Bodily Changes.* 4th ed. New York: Columbia University Press, 1954.

Dychtwald, Kenneth. *Bodymind.* New York: Jove Publications, 1977.

Ehrlich, Paul; Ehrlich, Anne; and Holdren, John. *Human Ecology.* San Francisco: W. H. Freeman, 1973.

Eibl-Eibesfeldt, I. *Love and Hate: The Natural History of Behavior Patterns.* New York: Holt, Rinehart & Winston, Inc., 1972.

Eliade, Mircea. *Patanjali and Yoga.* New York: Schocken Books, Inc., 1975.

Esdaile, James. *Hypnosis in Medicine and Surgery.* New York: Julian Press, 1957.

Evans-Wentz, W. Y. *The Tibetan Book of the Dead.* New York: Oxford University Press, 1960.

Fabrega, Horatio, Jr. *Disease and Social Behavior.* Cambridge, MA: The Massachusetts Institute of Technology Press, 1974.

———. The Need for an Ethnomedical Science. *Science,* 1975: 189, 969.

Faraday, Ann. *The Dream Game.* New York: Harper & Row Publishers, Inc., 1974.

Feifel, Herman. *New Meanings of Death.* New York: McGraw-Hill Book Co., 1977.

Feldenkrais, Moshe. *Awareness Through Movement.* New York: Harper & Row Publishers, Inc., 1972.

Ferguson, Marilyn. *Brain Revolution.* New York: Bantam Books, 1973.

———. *The Aquarian Conspiracy.* Los Angeles: J. P. Tarcher, 1980.

Ferguson, Tom, ed. *Medical Self-Care: Access to Medical Tools.* New York: Summit Books, 1979.

Fixx, James F. *The Complete Book of Running.* New York: London House, 1977.

Flammonde, Pavis. *The Mystic Healers.* New York: Stein & Day, 1974.

Fletcher, G. G., and Cantwell, J. D. *Exercise and Coronary Heart Disease.* Springfield, IL: Charles C Thomas, 1974.

Fosshage, James L., and Olsen, Paul, eds. *Healing: Implications for Psychotherapy.* New York: Human Sciences Press, Inc., 1978.

Frank, Jerome D. *Persuasion and Healing.* New York: Schocken Books, Inc., 1963.

Fuchs, Victor R. *Who Shall Live? Health Economics and Social Choice.* New York: Basic Books, Inc., 1974.

Garfield, Charles A. *Psychosocial Care of the Dying Patient.* New York: McGraw-Hill Book Co., 1978.

Gartner, Alan, and Reissman, Frank. *Self-Help in the Human Services.* San Francisco: Jossey-Bass Inc., Publishers, 1977.

Geba, B. H. *Breathe Away Your Tension.* New York: Random House, Inc., 1973.

Golas, Thaddeus. *The Lazy Man's Guide to Enlightenment.* Palo Alto, CA: The Seed Center, 1972.

Goldstein, Joseph. *The Experience of Insight: A Natural Unfolding.* Santa Cruz, CA: Unity Press, 1976.

Goodheart, G. *Applied Kinesiology Notes*. Detroit, MI: Author, 1972–1977.

Gordon, James; Jaffe, Dennis; and Bresler, David, eds. *Mind, Body, and Health: Toward an Integral Medicine*. Rockville, MD: National Institute of Mental Health, in press, 1982.

Govinda, L. A. *Creative Meditation and Multi-Dimensional Consciousness*. Wheaton, IL: Theosophical Publishing House, 1976.

———. *Way of the White Clouds*. Berkeley, CA: Shambhala Press, Inc., 1971.

Grant, Lillian. *The Holistic Revolution*. New York: Crown Publishers, Inc., 1978.

Green, Elmer, and Green, Alyce. *Beyond Feedback*. New York: Delta. 1977.

Grof, Stanislav. *Realms of the Human Unconscious, Observations from LSD Research*. New York: E. P. Dutton & Company, Inc., 1976.

Gunther, Bernard. *Sense Relaxation*. New York: Collier, 1968.

Gurdjieff, G. I. *Meetings with Remarkable Men*. New York: E. P. Dutton & Company, Inc., 1969.

Hahnemann, Samuel. *Organon of Medicine*. 6th ed. Translated by William Boericke. New Delhi: Harjeet, 1974.

Haley, Jay. *Uncommon Therapy: The Psychiatric Techniques of Milton H. Erickson*. New York: W. W. Norton & Co., Inc., 1973.

Halifax, Joan. *Shamanic Voices*. New York: E. P. Dutton & Company, Inc., 1979.

Hall, Robert K; Hall, Alyssa; Heckler, Catherine; and Heckler, Richard K. *The Lomi Papers*. Mill Valley, CA: Lomi School Press, 1975.

Hallowell, A. I. *Culture and Experience*. Philadelphia: University of Pennsylvania Press, 1955.

Halprin, Anna. *Movement Ritual*. San Francisco: Dancers' Workshop, 1979.

———. *Movement Ritual I*. San Francisco: Dancers' Workshop, 1975.

———. *Collected Writings I and II*. San Francisco: Dancers' Workshop, 1975.

———. *Exit to Enter*. Dancers' Workshop, 1973.

Halprin, Anna, and Burns, Jim. *As School Comes Home*. Los Angeles: Panjandrum Press, 1973.

Halprin, Anna; Nixon, James Hurd; and Burns, Jim. *Citydance 1977*. San Francisco: Dancers' Workshop, 1977.

Hastings, Arthur; Fadiman, James; and Gordon, James S. *Health for the Whole Person*. Boulder, CO: Westview Press, 1980.

Hill, Ann, ed. *A Visual Encyclopedia of Unconventional Medicine*. New York: Crown Publishers, Inc., 1979.

Himber, Jacob. *The Complete Family Guide to Dental Health*. New York: McGraw-Hill Book Company, 1977.

Hintz, Naomi, and Pratt, J. G. *The Psychic Realm: What Can We Believe?* New York: Random House, Inc., 1975.

Holzer, Hans. *Beyond Medicine*. New York: Ballantine Books, 1973.

Howard, B. *Dance of the Self*. New York: Simon & Schuster, Inc., 1974.

Hsu, Francis. *Psychological Anthropology*. Cambridge, MA: Schenkman Publishing Company, Inc., 1972.

Huard, Pierre, and Wong, Ming. *Chinese Medicine*. New York: McGraw-Hill Book Company, 1968.

Hutschnecker, Arnold. *The Will to Live*. New York: Cornerstone Library, Inc., 1975.

Huxley, Aldous. *The Perennial Philosophy*. New York: Harper & Row Publishers, Inc., 1970.

Ichazo, Oscar. *The Human Process for Enlightenment and Freedom*. New York: Arica Institute, Inc., 1976.

Illich, Ivan. *Medical Nemesis: the Expropriation of Health*. New York: Pantheon Books, 1976.

International Chiropractic Association. *Modern Developments in the Principles and Practice of Chiropractic*. New York: Appleton-Century-Crofts, 1979.

Ismael, Cristina. *The Healing Environment*. Millbrae, CA: Celestial Arts Publishing Co., 1976.

Jackson, Mildred, and Teague, Terri. *The Handbook of Alternatives to Chemical Medicine*. Oakland, CA: Lawton-Teague, 1975.

Jaffe, Dennis. *Healing from Within*. New York: Alfred A. Knopf, Inc., 1978.

James, Dorothy. *Politics, and Change*. Englewood Cliffs, NJ: Prentice-Hall, Inc., 1972.

Jones, F. P. *Body Awareness in Action*. New York: Schocken Books, Inc., 1976.

Journal of Holistic Health, Vol. III. San Diego, CA: The Word Shop, 1978.

Joy, W. Brugh. *Joy's Way*. Los Angeles: J. P. Tarcher, 1979.

Jung, Carl G. *Man and His Symbols*. New York: Doubleday & Company, Inc., 1964.

Jung, Carl G., with Jaffe, Aniela. *Memories, Dreams, Reflections*. New York: Vintage Books, 1965.

Kaplan, H. S. *The New Sex Therapy*. New York: Brunner/Mazel, Inc., 1974.

Kapleau, Philip. *The Three Pillars of Zen*. Boston: Beacon Press, Inc., 1967.

Karlins, M., and Andrews, L. *Biofeedback: Turning on the Power of Your Mind*. Philadelphia: J. B. Lippincott Co., 1972.

Kaslof, Leslie J., ed. *Wholistic Dimensions in Healing*. New York: Doubleday and Company, Inc., 1978.

Kastenbaum, Robert, and Aisenberg, Ruth. *The Psychology of Death*. New York: Springer Publishing, 1972.

Kennett, Roshi Jiyu. *How to Grow a Lotus Blossom*. Shasta Abbey of the Reformed Soto Zen Church, Mt. Shasta, CA 96067, 1977.

————. *Zen is Eternal Life*. Emeryville, CA: Dharma Publishing, 1976.

Kennett, Roshi Jiyu, and Macphillamy, Daizui. *The Book of Life*. Mt. Shasta, CA: Shasta Abbey Press, 1979.

Kiev, Ari. *Magic, Faith and Healing*. New York: Free Press, 1969.

————. *Transcultural Psychiatry*. New York: Free Press, 1972.

Kilner, Walter J. *The Aura*. New York: Samuel Weiser, Inc., 1973.

Kinnear, Willis, ed. *Spiritual Healing*. Los Angeles: Science of Mind Publications, 1973.

Koestler, Arthur. *The Roots of Coincidence*. New York: Vintage Books, 1973.

Kovel, Joel. *A Complete Guide to Therapy*. New York: Pantheon Books, 1976.

Kramer, Joel. *The Passionate Mind*. Millbrae, CA: Celestial Arts, Inc., 1974.

Krippner, Stanley. *Song of the Siren*. New York: Harper & Row Publishers, Inc., 1975.

Krippner, Stanley, and Rubin, Daniel, eds. *The Kirlian Aura*. New York: Anchor/Doubleday, 1974.

Krippner, Stanley, and Villoldo, Alberto. *The Realms of Healing*. Millbrae, CA: Celestial Arts, Inc., 1976.

Kruger, Helen. *Other Healers, Other Cures—A Guide to Alternative Medicine*. New York: Bobbs-Merrill Company, Inc., 1974.

Kubler-Ross, Elisabeth. *On Death and Dying*. New York: Macmillan Publishing Co., Inc. 1969.

Kuhn, Thomas S. *The Structure of Scientific Revolutions*. Chicago: University of Chicago Press, 1962.

Kurtz, Ron, and Prestera, Hector. *The Body Reveals*. New York: Bantam Books, Inc., 1976.

Laing, R. D. *The Politics of Experience*. New York: Ballantine Books, 1968.

Landy, David, ed. *Culture, Disease and Healing*. Macmillan Publishing Co., Inc., 1977.

Lappe, Frances M. *Diet for a Small Planet*. New York: Ballantine Books, Inc., 1975.

Laszlo, Ervin. *The Relevance of General Systems Theory.* New York: George Braziller, Inc., 1972.

Law, Donald. *A Guide to Alternative Medicine.* New York: Doubleday & Company, Inc., 1976.

Lazarus, R. *Patterns of Adjustment.* New York: McGraw-Hill Book Company, 1976.

Leadbeater, C. W. *The Chakras.* Wheaton, IL: The Theosophical Publishing House, 1927.

Leboyer, Frederick. *Birth Without Violence.* New York: Alfred A. Knopf, Inc., 1975.

Lecron, Leslie M. *Self Hypnotism.* Englewood Cliffs, NJ: Prentice-Hall, Inc., 1964.

———. *Techniques of Hypnotherapy.* New York: Julian Press, 1961.

Leonard, George. *The Transformation.* New York: Delacorte Press, 1972.

———. *The Ultimate Athlete.* New York: Viking Press, 1975.

Leonard, Jon N.; Hofer, J. L.; and Pritikin, Nathan. *Live Longer Now.* Grosset & Dunlap, 1976.

Leshan, Lawrence. *How to Meditate.* Cambridge, MA: Brown & Company, 1974.

———. *The Medium, the Mystic, and the Physicist.* New York: Viking Press, 1974.

Leslie, Charles, ed. *Asian Medical Systems: A Comparative Study.* Berkeley: University of California Press, 1976.

Levin, Lowell S.; Katz, Alfred H.; and Holst, Erik. *Self-Care: Lay Initiatives in Health.* New York: Prodist Press, 1976.

Lilly, John C. *The Center of the Cyclone.* New York: Bantam Books, Inc., 1972.

Lindemann, Hannes. *Relieve Tension the Autogenic Way.* New York: Peter H. Wyden, 1974.

Loomis, Evarts, and Paulson, J. *Healing for Everyone.* New York: Hawthorne Books, 1975.

Lowen, Alexander. *Pleasure.* New York: Penguin Books, 1976.

———. *Bioenergetics.* New York: Coward, McCann & Geoghegan, Inc., 1975.

———. *Depression and the Body.* New York: Penguin Books, 1972.

———. *The Language of the Body.* New York: Collier, 1971.

Luce, Gay. *Your Second Life.* New York: Seymour Lawrence/Delacorte, 1979.

———. *Body Time.* New York: Bantam Books, Inc., 1973.

————. *Biological Rhythms in Human and Animal Physiology.* New York: Dover Publications, Inc., 1971.

Luthe, W. *Autogenic Training.* New York: Grune & Stratton, 1965.

Luthe, W., and Schultz, J.H. *Autogenic Therapy, Vols. 1-6.* New York: Grune & Stratton, 1969.

Macnutt, Francis, O. P. *Healing.* Notre Dame, IN: Ave Maria Press, 1974.

Maigne, Robert. *Orthopedic Medicine.* Springfield, IL: Charles C Thomas, 1972.

Maltz, Maxwell. *Psychocybernetics.* North Hollywood, CA: Wilshire Book Company, 1965.

Mann, Felix. *Acupuncture—The Ancient Chinese Art of Healing and How It Works Scientifically.* New York: Random House, Inc., 1974.

————. *The Meridians of Acupuncture.* London: William Heinemann Medical Books, 1964.

Maslow, Abraham H. *Farther Reaches of Human Nature.* New York: Viking Press, 1971.

————. *Motivation and Personality.* 2d ed. New York: Harper & Row Publishers, Inc., 1970.

————. *Toward a Psychology of Being.* New York: Van Nostrand, 1968.

Masters, Robert, and Houston, Jean. *The Varieties of Psychedelic Experience.* New York: Dell Publishing Company, Inc., 1966.

Mattson, Phyllis. *Holistic Health in Perspective.* San Francisco: Institute of Noetic Sciences, 1978.

McGarey, William A. *Acupuncture and Body Energies.* Phoenix, AZ: Gabriel Press, 1974.

McKeown, Thomas. *The Role of Medicine: Dream, Mirage, or Nemesis?* London: Rock Carline Fellowship, Nuffield Provincial Hospitals Trust, 1976.

Mendelsohn, Robert S. *Confessions of a Medical Heretic.* New York: Warner Communications Company, 1979.

Middleton, J., ed. *Magic, Witchcraft and Curing.* Garden City, NY: Natural History Press, 1967.

Miller, Emmett M. *Feeling Good: How To Stay Healthy.* Englewood Cliffs, NJ: Prentice-Hall, Inc., 1978.

Millman, M. *The Unkindest Cut.* New York: William Morrow & Co., Inc., 1977.

Mitchell, Edgar. *Psychic Exploration.* John White, ed. New York: G. P. Putnam's Sons, 1974.

Montagu, Ashley. *Touching.* New York: Harper & Row Publishers, Inc., 1971.

Montgomery, Ruth. *Born To Heal*. New York: Popular Library, Inc., 1973.

Moody, Raymond. *Life After Life*. Atlanta, GA: Mockingbird Books, 1975.

Morehouse, L., and Gross, L. *Total Fitness*. New York: Simon & Schuster, Inc., 1975.

Mostofsky, D. I., ed. *Behavioral Control and the Modification of Physiological Processes*. Englewood Cliffs, NJ: Prentice-Hall, Inc., 1976.

Murphy, Michael, and White, Rhea. *The Psychic Side of Sports*. Reading, MA: Addison Wesley, 1978.

Nader, Laura, and Maretzki, Thomas W. *Cultural Illness and Health*. Washington, D.C.: American Anthropological Association, 1973.

Naranjo, Claudio, and Ornstein, Robert. *On the Psychology of Meditation*. New York: Viking Press, 1971.

National Council on Aging. *Facts and Myths About Aging*. Washington, D.C.: author, 1977.

Newbold, H. L. *Mega-Nutrients*. New York: Peter H. Wyden, 1975.

Nutrition Search, Inc. *Nutrition Almanac*. New York: McGraw-Hill Book Company, 1975.

Nyhan, William L. *The Heredity Factor*. New York: Grosset & Dunlap, 1976.

Ohashi, Watari. *Do-It-Yourself Shiatsu: Japanese Acupressure*. New York: E. P. Dutton, 1976.

Ornstein, Robert. *The Mind Field*. New York: Grossman Publishers, 1976.

———. *Psychology of Consciousness*. San Francisco: W. H. Freeman & Company, 1972.

Otto, Herbert A., and Knight, James W., eds. *Dimensions in Wholistic Healing: New Frontiers in the Treatment of the Whole Person*. Chicago: Nelson-Hall, Inc., 1979.

Otto, Herbert A., and Mann, J. *Ways of Growth*. New York: Viking Press, 1968.

Ouspensky, P. D. *In Search of the Miraculous*. New York: Harcourt, Brace, Jovanovich, Inc., 1965.

Oyle, Irving. *The Healing Mind*. Millbrae, CA: Celestial Arts, Inc., 1975.

———. *Time, Space and the Mind*. Millbrae, CA: Celestial Arts, Inc., 1976.

Page, I. H. *The Cholesterol Fallacy*. Cleveland, OH: Coronary Club, 1977.

Palos, Stephen. *The Chinese Art of Healing*. New York: McGraw-Hill Book Company, 1971.

Parsons, Talcott. *The Social System*. New York: Free Press, 1951.

Pauling, Linus. *Vitamin C and the Common Cold*. San Francisco: W. H. Freeman & Company, 1970.

Pearce, Joseph Chilton. *Crack in the Cosmic Egg*. New York: Pocket Books, 1974.

Pelletier, Kenneth R. *Holistic Medicine, from Stress to Optimum Health*. New York: Delacorte Press, 1979.

———. *Mind as Healer, Mind as Slayer*. New York: Delacorte Press, 1977.

———. *Toward a Science of Consciousness*. New York: Delacorte Press, 1978.

Peper, Erik, et al., eds. *Mind/Body Integration: Essential Readings in Biofeedback*. New York: Plenum Press, 1978.

Perls, Fritz. *Gestalt Therapy Verbatim*. Lafayette, IN: Real People Press, 1969.

Pfeiffer, Carl C. *Mental and Elemental Nutrients: A Physician's Guide to Nutrition and Health Care*. New Canaan, CT: Keats Publishing Company, 1975.

Pirsig, R. M. *Zen and the Art of Motorcycle Maintenance*. New York: Bantam Books, Inc., 1974.

Popenoe, Cris. *Wellness*. Washington, D.C.: Yes! Inc., 1977.

Porkert, Manfred. *The Theoretical Foundations of Chinese Medicine*. Cambridge: Massachusetts Institute of Technology Press, 1974.

Porter, Jean. *Psychic Development*. New York: Random House, Inc., 1974.

Proshansky, Harold M., et al. *Environmental Psychology: People and Their Physical Settings*. New York: Holt, Rinehart & Winston, Inc., 1976.

Rabkin, Richard. *Inner and Other Space: Introduction to a Theory of Social Psychiatry*. New York: W. W. Norton & Co., Inc., 1970.

Ram Dass. *The Only Dance There Is*. New York: Anchor Press, 1974.

Ram Dass, and Levine, Stephen. *Grist for the Mill*. Santa Cruz, CA: Unity Press, 1977.

Rechung, Jampal Kunzang Rinpoche. *Tibetan Medicine*. Berkeley: University of California Press, 1973.

Reich, Wilhelm. *Selected Writings*. New York: Noonday Press, 1973.

Reiser, Stanley Joel. *Medicine and The Reign of Technology*. New York: Cambridge University Press, 1978.

Remen, Naomi. *The Human Patient*. Garden City, NY: Anchor/Doubleday, 1980.

———. *The Masculine Principle, the Feminine Principle and Humanistic Medicine*. San Francisco: Institute for the Study of Humanistic Medicine, 1975.

Risse, Guenter B.; Numbers, Ronald A.; and Leavitt, Judith Walzer. *Medicine Without Doctors*. New York: Science History Publications, 1977.

Rolf, Ida P. *Rolfing*. Santa Monica, CA: Dennis Landman, 1977.

Rush, A. K. *Getting Clear: Body Work for Women*. New York: Random House, Inc., 1973.

Rutstein, David. *The Coming Revolution in Medicine*. Cambridge: The Massachusetts Institute of Technology Press, 1967.

Salk, Jonas. *Survival of the Wisest*. New York: Harper & Row Publishers, Inc., 1973.

———. *Man Unfolding*. R. N. Anshen, ed. New York: Harper & Row Publishers, Inc., 1972.

Samuels, M., and Samuels, N. *Seeing with the Mind's Eye*. New York: Random House, Inc., 1973.

Samuels, Mike, and Bennett, Hal. *The Well Body Book*. New York: Random House, Inc., 1973.

Sannella, Lee. *Kundalini—Psychosis or Transcendence?* San Francisco: H. S. Dakin Company, 1978.

Satin, Mark. *New Age Politics: Healing Self and Society*. West Vancouver, B.C.: Whitecap Books, 1978.

Satir, Virginia. *Peoplemaking*. Palo Alto, CA: Science and Behavior Books, 1972.

Saward, Ernest. The Current Emphasis on Preventive Medicine. *Science*, 200: 889-894.

Schumacher, E. F. *Small is Beautiful*. New York: Harper & Row Publishers, Inc., 1976.

Schwartz, G., and Shapiro, D., eds. *Consciousness and Self-Regulation*. New York: Plenum Press, 1976.

Schwartz, Gary E., and Beatty, J., eds. *Biofeedback, Theory and Research*. New York: Academic Press, 1978.

Seligman, A. A. *Helplessness*. San Francisco: W. H. Freeman, 1975.

Selye, Hans. *Stress Without Distress*. New York: E. P. Dutton, 1974.

———. *The Stress of Life*. New York: McGraw-Hill Book Company, 1956.

Shapiro, Deane. *Precision Nirvana*. Englewood Cliffs, NJ: Prentice-Hall, Inc., 1977.

Shealy, C. Norman. *The Pain Game*. Millbrae, CA: Celestial Arts, Inc., 1976.

———. *Ninety Days to Self-Health*. New York: Dial Press, 1977.

Sherman, Ingrid. *Natural Remedies for Better Health*. Happy Camp, CA: Naturegraph Publishers, Inc., 1970.

Sigerist, H. Primitive and Archaic Medicine. *A History of Medicine. Vol. I*. London: Oxford University Press, 1951.

Simonton, O.C.: Matthews-Simonton, S.; and Creighton, J. *Getting Well Again.* Los Angeles: J.P. Tarcher, 1978.

Smith, David. *The East-West Exercise Book.* New York: McGraw-Hill Book Company, 1976.

Smith, M. Brewster. Humanism and Behaviorism in Psychology, Theory and Practice. *Journal of Humanistic Psychology,* Vol. 18, No. 1, Winter 1978.

Smuts, Jan Christiaan. *Holism and Evolution.* New York: Macmillan Publishing Co., Inc., 1926.

Sobel, David S. *Ways of Health: Holistic Approaches to Ancient and Contemporary Medicine.* New York: Harcourt, Brace, Jovanovich, Inc., 1979.

Sobel, David S. and Hornbacher, F.L. *An Everyday Guide to Your Health.* New York: Grossman, 1973.

Somers, Anne R. *Health Care in Transition: Directions for the Future.* Chicago: Hospital Research and Educational Trust, 1971.

Sontag, Susan. *Illness as Metaphor.* New York: Farrar, Straus & Giroux, 1978.

Spangler, David. *Revelation: The Birth of a New Age.* Findhorn, Scotland: The Findhorn Foundation, 1971.

Speads, Carola H. *Breathing, The ABC's.* New York. Harper & Row Publishers, Inc., 1978.

————. Physical Re-education: What It Is and What It Is Not. *Somatics Magazine—Journal of the Bodily Arts and Sciences,* Vol. 1, No. 2, Spring, 1977.

Stapleton, Ruth. *The Experience of Inner Healing.* New York: Word, Inc., 1976.

Stransky, Judith, with Stone, Robert B. *The Alexander Technique.* New York: Beaufort Books, Inc., 1981.

Swami Rama. *A Practical Guide to Holistic Health.* Honesdale, PA: Himalayan International Institute, 1978.

Swami Rama; Ballentine, Rudolph; and Hymes, Alan. *Science of Breath, A Practical Guide.* Honesdale, PA: Himalayan International Institute, 1979.

Tager, Mark, and Jennings, Charles. *Whole Person Health.* Portland, OR: Victoria House Publishers, 1978.

Tart, Charles T. *States of Consciousness.* New York: E.P. Dutton, 1975.

————. *Altered States of Consciousness.* New York: John Wiley & Sons, Inc., 1969.

Thie, John F. D. C. *Touch for Health*. Santa Monica, CA: Devorss & Company, 1973.

Thomas, L. *The Lives of a Cell*. New York: Bantam Books, Inc., 1975.

Travis, John W. *Wellness Workbook*. Mill Valley, CA: Wellness Resource Center, 1975.

Trungpa, Chogyam. *Cutting Through Spiritual Materialism*. Berkeley, CA: Shambala Press, 1973.

———. *Meditation in Action*. Berkeley, CA: Shambhala Press, 1969.

Tubesing, Donald A. *The Wholistic Health Center*. New York: Human Sciences Press, 1979.

Tulku, T. *Reflections of the Mind*. Berkeley, CA: Dharma Press, 1975.

Turner, Victor. *The Forest of Symbols*. Ithaca, NY: Cornell University Press, 1967.

———. *The Ritual Process*. Chicago: Aldine Publishing Company, 1969.

Veith, Ilza, trans. *The Yellow Emperor's Classic of Internal Medicine*. Berkeley: University of California Press, 1972.

Vickery, D. M. and Fries, J. F. *Take Care of Yourself: A Consumer's Guide to Medical Care*. Reading, MA: Addison-Wesley, 1977.

Virchow, R. *Disease, Life and Man*. Stanford, CA: Stanford University Press, 1978.

Vithoulklas, George. *The Science of Homeopathy, a Modern Text*. Athens, Greece: Athens School of Homeopathic Medicine, 1978.

———. *Homeopathy: Medicine of the New Man*. New York: Avon Books, 1972.

Vogel, Virgil J. *American Indian Medicine*. Norman: University of Oklahoma Press, 1970.

Wade, Carlson. *Health Secrets from the Orient*. Englewood, NJ: Parker Publishing Company, 1973.

Wallace, Amy, and Henkin, Bill. *The Psychic Healing Book*. New York: Delacorte Press, 1978.

Walther, David S. *Applied Kinesiology, Volume I—Basic Procedures and Muscle Testing*. Pueblo, CO: Systems DC, 1981.

———. *Applied Kinesiology Flow Chart*. Pueblo, CO: Systems DC, 1980.

———. *Applied Kinesiology*. Pueblo, CO: Systems DC, 1978.

———. *Applied Kinesiology Programmed Instruction* (10 volumes). Pueblo, CO: Systems DC, 1977-1978.

———. *Applied Kinesiology—The Advanced Approach in Chiropractic*. Pueblo, CO: Systems DC, 1976.

Watson, George. *Nutrition and Your Mind: The Psychochemical Response.* New York: Harper & Row Publishers, Inc., 1972.

Watts, Alan. *The Way of Zen.* New York: Pantheon Books, 1967.

Wells, L. *Kinesiology.* Philadelphia: W. B. Saunders Co., 1955.

Wheelis, A. *How People Change.* New York: Harper & Row Publishers, Inc., 1973.

White, J. *The Highest State of Consciousness.* New York: Doubleday & Co., Inc., 1972.

Williams, Roger. *The Wonderful World Within You: Your Inner Nutritional Environment.* New York: Bantam Books, 1977.

———. *Nutrition Against Disease.* New York: Bantam Books, 1973.

———. *Nutrition in a Nutshell.* New York: Dolphin Books, 1962.

Williams, Roger, and Kalita, Dwight, eds. *A Physicians's Handbook on Orthomolecular Medicine.* Elmsford, NY: Pergamon Press, 1977.

Worrall, Ambrose, and Worrall, Olga. *The Gift of Healing.* New York: Harper & Row Publishers, Inc., 1965.

Worsley, Jack. *The Meridians of Ch'i Energy: Point Reference Guide.* Great Britain, 1979.

———. *Is Acupuncture for You?* New York: Harper & Row Publishers, Inc., 1973.

Wu, Shui Wan. *The Chinese Pulse Diagnosis.* Los Angeles: author, 1972.

Yogananda, Paramahansa. *The Autobiography of a Yogi.* Los Angeles: Self-Realization Fellowship, 1977.

INDEX

C

I

J

K

0 0 4 4 0 4 0

HOLISTIC MEDICINE HA
RMONY OF BODY